DATE DUE		

A LITTLE WORK

A LITTLE WORK

Behind the Doors of a Park Avenue Plastic Surgeon

Z. PAUL LORENC,
M.D., F.A.C.S.

AND TRISH HALL

ST. MARTIN'S PRESS

NEW YORK

www.stmartins.com

ISBN 0-312-31524-4
EAN 978-0312-31524-5

10 9 8 7 6 5 4 3 2

This book is dedicated to my mother and father,
whose faith, strength, and courage shaped my future.

—Z.P.L.

A NOTE TO READERS

CONTENTS

ACKNOWLEDGMENTS

To my wife, Lorraine, with grateful affection for enriching my life with her vision, energy, enthusiasm, and companionship. And to our two children, who make every day worthwhile. To my teachers Sherrell Aston, Dan Baker, and Tom Rees, special thanks for guiding my discovery of the art and science of aesthetic plastic surgery.

—Z.P.L.

This book exists only because of the hard work and extraordinary humor of my agent, Alice Martell. And although I'd like to thank all of my friends and family for their encouragement and support, I could not possibly have written this, or anything else, without my husband, Larry Wolhandler, and my daughter, Hally.

—T.H.

A LITTLE WORK

One

A DAY IN THE LIFE

6 A.M.

THERE ARE MORNING PEOPLE AND THERE ARE NIGHT PEOPLE. I GUESS I'm both.

Lucky for me, I don't need a lot of sleep. And I always wake up eager to start the day.

I love the timer on the coffeemaker. When I get out of bed, I can grab a cup before jumping in the shower. I watch the news on the small TV in the bathroom as I shave, figure out which suit and tie to wear—in my business, image is crucial—then get dressed, talk to Lorraine, who also manages the office, about the logistics of the day, then kiss the kids, Paul and Christina, good-bye. They're almost always still sleeping when I leave.

6:45 A.M.

It is a crisp, ice-blue Monday in December, and by the time I walk out the door of my town house on the Upper East Side of Manhattan, there is only one thing on my mind: surgery. Monday is one of my surgery days, and I'm scheduled to operate on Rebecca, a woman in her early fifties who is unhappy with both the way her eyes look, especially how droopy her lids have become, and the deep lines etched on her forehead.

I practice on Park Avenue and operate both in my office and at Manhattan Eye, Ear and Throat (also just called Manhattan Eye and Ear), the hospital where some of the best-known doctors in the field also do their surgeries. I see men and women, young people and old people. They're not like Michael Jackson. They don't want new faces.

They want *their* faces. Only better.

Plastic surgery was once the province of the rich or famous, and of wealthy women in their sixties and seventies, but no more. Over the course of my sixteen years in practice, I've seen the average age drop by about two decades. Now people are coming in for face-lifts in their forties and early fifties. The economic range is vast too. One of my patients is a teacher's aide who makes $12,000 a year. Another has houses all over the world and traveled to New York from her primary residence in London for a total body sculpting before going on to her house in the Caribbean to recuperate. In just the last five years it has become an international business, especially for New York doctors. We had a sultan with ten wives come for liposuction. Not an entirely easy process. When he came for follow-up care and he couldn't get his compression garment back on, my assistant had to dress him without looking at him or touching him, since women outside his family weren't allowed to do either of those things. Sultans or schoolteachers, they find a way to pay for it if they want it.

As much as I love surgery, I am also entranced by meeting with new patients. I see every possible kind of complaint and hear every possible kind of request. I see young women who have the tiniest flaws in their faces that to them seem enormous, and as silly as it would seem to an outsider, they are convinced that their happiness depends on correcting them. I see women who have breasts so large that they live with debilitating, chronic back pain from supporting them, and when they have their breasts reduced, they feel physically comfortable for the first time in their adult lives.

And, sad to say, I see lots of other plastic surgeons' mistakes. Their unhappy patients want to start over, to go back to their original faces. Unfortunately, that can rarely happen.

But I'm not thinking about mistakes right now. I go over Rebecca's face in my mind, visualizing exactly what I will be doing later in the morning. The patient, a teacher with long gray-streaked brown hair and a vivid smile, is getting a brow-lift to smooth out her forehead, and a blepharoplasty, which is the procedure to cut out the fat and the excess skin from her upper eyelids. I'll be doing the procedure in a fully equipped and accredited surgical suite in my office.

First I'll finish her upper lid, a procedure that takes only thirty minutes and will open up her eyes, leaving a nearly invisible scar in the crease of her lid. Next comes the endoscopic brow-lift. With this technique, I make two small incisions in her hairline above her forehead. With instruments connected to a camera and a computer, I work on the muscles in her forehead so that her eyebrows can return to their original position. When I finish, she will look as if someone has slightly lifted her forehead and thinned out her eyelids. Not radically different, but better. Rested, more alert.

The surgery will take about two hours. After, she'll look pretty bloody, because the eyes ooze, and obviously there's no way to completely bandage them so that nothing shows. The incisions in her hair for the brow-lift won't be visible, but the hair around them will be matted, so she definitely won't be in the mood for socializing. She will have to have someone pick her up and take her home, and she'll spend most of that first day sleeping. When she isn't sleeping, she can put cold compresses on her eyes to make them feel better, but she won't need painkillers for the eyes. The brow-lift is another matter. That sometimes hurts, most often like a headache, and we recommend Vicodan if it does. She will come back to see me tomorrow to make sure all is well.

It will be perfectly routine and routinely perfect. I was one of the pioneers in developing the endoscopic brow-lift and can do it in my sleep. Still, I always like to think about things before I do them. I'm a big believer in visualization. Skiers use it, and so do baseball players. That's why I like to walk before I do surgery. By the time I have covered the nine blocks and arrive at my office, I have already performed, in my mind, every step of the surgery.

7 A.M.

I'm always the first person in the office. I walk in and turn on the lights. I move the skin-care creams that the staff left on the counter in the reception area. I hate to see clutter sitting there. When I am happy with the way everything looks, I go into my office and get out Rebecca's folder to take one last look. Before surgery, I never eat breakfast.

Last night, I reviewed the photos taken by a professional photographer about a week earlier. They showed every little pore on Rebecca's face, which is what I want. I have already marked up the photos with a pen, making the cuts with ink that I will later make with a scalpel. Basically, I draw the surgery, and sometimes I think that's the hardest, most important part of my job. If I make a mistake here, I will likely make a mistake in the operating room, and that isn't something I can erase.

I love surgery. I love doing surgery. I love thinking about surgery.

It's amazing to me to be given the trust that my patients offer. They don't come to me with an illness, or suffering or desperate. They are healthy people, often with fine-looking faces, who want simply to be restored to an image of themselves that makes them happy. Not necessarily to youth, but to what seems to them their true selves. Sometimes I treat people who have had cancerous lesions removed from their faces, and I am reconstructing their faces to save them from having a terrible defect. But usually, the work I do is subtle. Medically speaking, it is unnecessary. The faith my patients have that I will not hurt them is awe-inspiring.

7:30 A.M.

Satisfied with my plan, I gather up the photos and head back to change into my scrubs. I do procedures on younger, healthier people in my office, and tend to use the hospital for the more complex or riskier cases, usually due to a patient's age and medical condition.

I go through the door that separates the waiting and examining rooms into the surgical area. In the anteroom at a small stainless-steel sink, I wash my hands with antibacterial soap and put on the green scrubs I always wear. While I am at the sink, Lolita, who has been my scrub nurse for sixteen years, and Tim, the anesthesiologist I frequently work with, arrive. Lolita is very easygoing, a Filipino who is serious and quiet in the operating room yet anything but out of it. She can read my mind—I never even have to tell her what instrument I want. Tim is a perfectionist who has never given a patient too little or too much anesthesia. We enjoy working together.

We go into the operating room to set up the instruments, and by the time we're done, the patient has arrived, in a gown and ready to go. While Tim explains to her what drugs he will use and what effect they will have, I start marking her forehead and eyes with the lines that will guide the scalpel. We are all friendly, but calm and serious. Only when the patient is out do I put on the music, loud—one of my favorite All-man Brothers songs, to start with—and begin the socializing and bantering with my colleagues that is typical of surgical suites everywhere. When I make the first cuts, I am quiet—I need total concentration—but otherwise you'd think we were in any office. We talk about our kids and the movies we've seen—and of course office politics.

Sewing up Rebecca's forehead is the most time-consuming part of her brow-lift. When we are done, I can already tell that she will get a good result. There's nothing that makes me happier. Afterward, I am totally psyched, as usual. Surgery is such a high for me. When I walk out of there, I'm the happiest that I ever feel.

I do big procedures, like face-lifts, abdominoplasties, and brow-lifts, like this one, on Mondays and Fridays. Generally, Tuesdays, Wednesdays, and Thursdays are devoted to minor procedures like applying Botox and other injectible substances to smooth out lines in the face, to follow-up visits with patients after surgery, and to meeting with potential patients.

For the next few hours, it's time to see my patients.

Noon

Before I start, I stop into my private office to check e-mail and to answer phone calls from other doctors and from patients. When I finish, I wander into the small kitchen behind our reception area. It holds a wall of folders with patient records from the last two years, a small refrigerator and microwave, and a table where we eat lunch. I always eat lunch at twelve, usually a salad with grilled chicken. The kitchen is where I can really talk with my employees, out of earshot of our patients. This is the office world that the patients never see. They're meant to experience only the beautiful and comforting side of plastic surgery—the fresh orchid on the reception counter, the Louise Nevelson statue (modern art is one of my true passions), the custom-made chairs so lushly enveloping that no one wants to get up out of them, the carpet custom woven with softly swirling yellows and greens. The doctor in his expensive Italian-tailored Canali suit. The receptionist who is always smiling and who can be trusted never to discuss anything remotely confidential if any patients are sitting in the waiting room.

Not the endless paperwork, not the spilled coffee, and certainly not the arguments.

12:45 P.M.

I am nursing a cup of coffee when Lorraine comes in and grabs the mug out of my hands. She can do that because she's my wife. But most of the time, there is nothing during the workday to suggest that we are anything but colleagues, and I like it that way. It's part of having a professionally run office. At work, she goes by her original name, Lorraine Russo. Many of the patients don't know we're married, and unless we become quite friendly, or they ask, we see no reason to tell them.

I am still wearing my green scrubs, and my mask is hanging down limply beneath my chin.

"Get out there," she orders. "The patient in Room One has been sitting there for fifteen minutes."

It is going to be a very busy afternoon, and I know I have to listen to her if I'm not going to fall too far behind. Lorraine makes the trains run on time. I don't talk to patients about costs, or discounts, or insurance, or scheduling. I think only about the work that has to be done for the patient, because that's my focus.

December is always hectic in the plastic surgery world. People who want to change their faces or their bodies often do surgery around the holidays, because they have time off from work, time to hide out.

However, my time to hide out is apparently over, so I go back to my office and change into a suit and tie. I meet with patients in scrubs only if it can't be avoided. It's been difficult for me to come around to this position, but this is an image business, and it's important that I look my best.

Outside of Room 1, I straighten my tie, mentally preparing myself. Not steeling myself, because there are really very few patients I dislike. Whenever I meet a patient for the first time, it's like a first date, with the need to charm, to make someone happy. Most people don't *have* to come for plastic surgery, which means they certainly aren't going to hire a doctor they don't like, or with whom they feel no rapport, to open up and lift their breasts or shoot foreign substances into their faces. Many of my patients are trying to correct flaws that to some others are not noticeable, and this tends to mean they can be somewhat obsessive. But they can see what is real and what is not. As long as they understand what I can do for them and don't have unreasonable expectations, I am happy to work with them.

I meet all kinds of people, and most of them, I like. But if someone is really driving me crazy for whatever reason, I'll step out for a minute and give Lorraine a signal. She'll come in and tell me that "Dr. Robin" is on the phone, and I'll make my escape. But mostly, I enjoy my patients, and I especially like the fact that our relationship can continue over many years. Someone who starts out with Botox might get her breasts enlarged later and then, maybe in her forties, a face-lift.

12:48 P.M.

Janine is sitting nervously on the examining table, and I chat to ease her nerves, about the snow and about how I have just come back from Montego Bay, where the temperature was in the balmy seventies. I can see from her chart that she has a medical, not cosmetic, need for my help. She has skin cancer. Her surgery is scheduled for next week. During that procedure, called Mohs after the doctor who developed it, her dermatologist will take out the cancerous tissue and have it immediately analyzed by the pathologist. He will keep cutting until there is no evidence of any cancer, and then the patient will come to me right afterward for reconstruction.

For me, it's a satisfyingly complex procedure, like a jigsaw puzzle. I'll do a modified face-lift, turning the skin and covering the defect created by cutting out the cancer, so that no skin grafts are required. Essentially, the patient's excess skin is used to cover up the hole.

Looking at Janine's chart, I recall that she is the mother of a movie star. Not surprising. But stars aren't the backbone of my practice. For me, my best patients aren't the actresses and singers and well-known businessmen I've treated. The patient who brings in the most business is the one who plays bridge with her friends and tells everyone in sight that she went to Paul Lorenc, and he was great.

I find it very gratifying to give patients what they want. I don't tell people they need to change, but if they say they're unhappy, and they want guidance, I give it to them. They may not "need" surgery, at least not from another person's point of view, but it's their point of view that matters. If I think I can help them, they're not crazy, and the procedure they want is aesthetically reasonable as well as medically safe, I'll do it.

I explain the procedure to Janine and see some of the worry leave her face.

1:28 P.M.

I go to the kitchen to fill out her chart while the notes, which are needed both for my records and for my malpractice carrier, are still fresh. At a required seminar held by my malpractice carrier not long ago, all of the surgeons were told to practice medicine assuming that every patient who walks in will sue. It's a horrible way to think, and I hate thinking about it that way. But I have to make the notes, and see, of course, what is going on in the office.

Janine goes to talk to Lorraine. All of the patients interested enough to consider the next step have a brief meeting with her. She knows how they feel and what they are thinking about, because she has had surgery herself—which I did, of course, although some may think it a bit creepy to operate on your family. I don't agree. I like doing it because then I know they're getting the best possible outcome.

If patients request it, Lorraine shows them the leather-bound books filled with photographs of work I've done. But photographs can be doctored, and they can be deceiving. They really should be used only to give a sense of how I view the world.

At the end of their conversation, Lorraine tells the patient what the procedure will cost. The price is higher if it is done in the hospital, less if done in the operating room that is part of my office. Sometimes she cuts the price a little for friends and relatives. As I said, I'm not interested in talking about the money. I don't, and I won't. If a patient says she's poor and she needs a break on the cost of the Botox, I tell her to talk to Lorraine. She's been my office manager from the beginning; she was my first employee, shortly after I started my practice sixteen years ago, in 1988, and she has done everything around here, even work as a circulating nurse during surgery. We're a real team.

Some patients come in for consultations, pay $200 to talk to me and have all their questions answered, and then go away. Forever. I never see them again, and I never know whether they decided they just didn't want surgery, or whether they felt more comfortable with another doctor.

Some of them, on the other hand, book their procedures right away. Once they have made up their minds to come in, they can hardly wait to get it done. Others fall somewhere in the middle: they need to come back another time with more questions before they really commit. And sometimes, they set the surgery date and change it a few times, because on some level they're nervous or doubtful.

Or both.

1:35 P.M.

My next consultation is with a woman who works for a city agency and wants to have her breasts reduced. She is in her early forties, African American, a little overweight, appealingly direct and no-nonsense in her manner. She is wearing a 40 DDD bra. Her breasts are enormous, four or five times the size of a B-cup. She says she picked a surgeon by asking all of her friends who'd had breast work to show her the results. She liked what I did on one of her friends, and now here she is. Some of her other friends, she says, have never gotten back sensation in their nipples, and she doesn't want that to happen to her. She has to pay for the surgery herself, but because she is a city employee with good insurance, she is covered for the hospital costs, so it is possible for her to have it done.

She schedules her surgery with Lorraine for the following week.

1:50 P.M.

Next is Julia, a woman who has taken the train in from the suburbs, wanting to have her breasts enlarged. She is slim, in her early thirties, with long blond hair streaked with perfect highlights, big green eyes, and a very large diamond on her left hand. When I ask her to open her robe, it is easy to see why she is here.

"Your breasts used to be bigger, didn't they?" I say.

"They sure did," Julia replies. "Now they've shrunk and are all saggy from breast-feeding my two children."

I explain to her that post-breast-feeding droopiness is common, and that the solution is fairly simple. I can put in implants, and at the same time I can give her a mastoplexy, essentially a breast-lift. The skin is tightened, and the breast returns to the position it was in years before.

She listens carefully, nodding her head. "Don't you have something to show me?" she asks.

I'm puzzled for a moment, then I realize what she means. "Oh, an implant." I go to the cabinet and pull out the implant I use, but it doesn't really tell anyone much.

"This is made of silicone, and essentially it's just like a bag," I say. "I make a cut in your body and put it under the muscle of your breast. That way it won't move out of place. Once it is in the right location, I fill it with saline. The patient is placed in a sitting position by the anesthesiologist and I make sure it looks right. If it's too big or too little, I can make adjustments."

That's the beauty of the saline implants. The old silicone ones, apart from the health controversy and women claiming to have developed autoimmune diseases as a result, were one size, and that was it. There was no room for maneuvering during surgery. I tell her, too, that after our meeting Lorraine will show her photographs of implants I have put in.

"Don't look at them as a guide," I say. "Don't say I want this one but not this one. Just look at them as a reflection of my aesthetic judgment and how well I perform the surgery."

Julia emphasizes that she isn't looking for large breasts, which doesn't surprise me. Very few of my patients are. Based on her build and chest size, I tell her that she can handle large breasts, but that I assume she wants nothing bigger than a large B. She wants to know when she can exercise again, which is a common question from my patients. I think I've had only four or five patients in the last few years who haven't asked that question. They all seem to belong to gyms and to exercise regularly. She seems satisfied with that and goes to see Lorraine.

2:15 P.M.

Directly after Julia is Patricia, who, oddly enough, is another young blond mother from the suburbs. She, too, is an A cup wanting breast implants. And she, too, is the epitome of a wealthy suburban woman, carrying a Chanel purse on her shoulder and wearing a Prada suit. This isn't business attire, because she, like Julia, does not have a job.

Only afterward do I find out from Lorraine that Julia and Patricia are best friends. If they decide to do the surgery, they want to have a close friend to help them through it psychologically, someone who really understands.

Although it's not unusual for two women to want to share the experience, there are still people who keep every little procedure totally secret, or at least they try to. I'm not sure why. Maybe they don't want to deal with the disapproval, because there is still some in our society, although, given how much people talk about plastic surgery now, less than in years past. For those who disapprove, it's as if anyone who dares to improve his or her appearance is somehow cheating, or unfairly gaining an edge in the aging sweepstakes. Some people seem to think that certain procedures are okay, such as doing reconstructive work after cancer surgery, but others, such as face-lifts, are not. That it's okay to play God in some situations, but not in others. I don't really understand that kind of thinking, but there it is.

I don't judge any of my patients. You can't want to be a plastic surgeon and have a judgmental attitude about how your patients regard themselves. If they want to do something to improve their appearance, as long as it is appropriate and medically feasible (and, of course, not a risk), and they can afford it, then they should do it.

2:30 P.M.

I meet with Regina, a tough young woman with curly black hair. I recently lifted and enlarged her breasts, changing them from a saggy A cup to a nicely rounded B cup. Now, however, they are covered with a nasty red rash. She has developed an allergic reaction to Bacitracin, an over-the-counter antibiotic ointment that I recommend to reduce the chance of infection. She has been using it only on the incisions, as directed, but the rash has spread all over her breasts. She was very stoic and hadn't called me until it was unbearably itchy.

I tell her that if something like that happens again, she should call me right away. I could have helped her on the phone and spared her some misery. I always tell patients they can call me anytime, that no problem is too small or too trivial. I am there to help them.

The only thing I don't give out is my cell phone number, but they can always reach someone who can reach me. Regina can't really explain why she didn't call sooner. She is very mysterious about who she is and what she does. I think she could have continued to tolerate the itching, but she came in because she was worried that something had gone wrong with the implant.

I prescribe a steroid cream to clear up the rash and tell her to promise to call me if she has any other problems or questions.

2:45 P.M.

Next I see a good-looking man, David, in his late fifties. With swept-back silver hair and a sleek suit, you would think he is an investment banker, but actually he is a landscaper. He is scheduled to have surgery for a malignancy on his face that doesn't look like much, but something that looks minor can easily, when removed, leave a rather large hole. He will have the Mohs procedure and then several hours later, groggy and bandaged up, meet me at the hospital for facial reconstruction.

People think cosmetic and reconstructive surgery are two different worlds, but they really aren't. The patients cross over. I see it time and time again. After the medical problem is taken care of, patients often come back for cosmetic surgery. David might be one of them. He has been involved with landscaping some of the area's most opulent properties, and is very rich, but appealingly low key.

People like David are a pleasure to deal with. They are very direct partly because of their circumstances. They need plastic surgery, and there's no talking and thinking and deliberating about whether they should have it.

They're the easy patients.

Unlike my next one.

3:00 P.M.

From the minute I walk into Room 2, I can tell Jolinda is really mad.

She is from the Bronx, with a face that was once beautiful but is start-ing to look hard and a little angry at age forty-two. She originally came to me because she was having trouble with her husband, and she wanted bigger breasts as a way to reignite their marriage. I did the surgery, and now, a year later, she is back because the implants have become hard.

Apparently they had also failed to save her marriage.

Jolinda has gotten what is called a capsule, which is the hard scar tis-sue that forms around the implant. In the course of my practice, I inevitably get patients who are unhappy about something. It doesn't happen frequently, but it happens. Jolinda is convinced that I could have or should have done something differently, that I somehow gave her bad advice on the follow-up care.

"My girlfriend had them at the same time from a different doctor and she didn't get a capsule because she massaged them every day," she says. "Why didn't you tell me to massage my breast like my friend's doctor did?"

There is no scientific proof, I tell her, that massage works. A capsule is just something that happens to some people, and there is no way to pre-dict its occurrence. "Massage might make them feel better, but it doesn't actually do anything about the capsule," I try to explain.

I have seen only two other capsules in sixteen years of practice, both of them from mistakes right after surgery. In the first case, the patient had a large one-year-old child, and right after surgery she called and said she heard something crunch or snap inside when she picked up her child. It wasn't until four or five years later that the implant actually hardened.

In the other case, a nurse made a mistake. Directly after surgery, patients are supposed to be picked up from the back so the implants are not disturbed. This nurse pulled the woman up out of bed by the arms, and the patient got a hematoma, a large bruise. I was able to fix it right away. But I also made it clear to the nurse that by being so careless she had forced a patient to go through a second surgical procedure.

But now Jolinda is sitting on the examining table, seething. She obviously believes that the problem was my fault. I try to explain the science to her—that a scar naturally forms around any implant, because the implant is an invader, an object not part of the body. In most people, the scar is small and not noticeable. But in some, it is large, and there is no way to predict it or avoid it. I tell her that the implant will have to come out and a new one put in.

When she hears that, her face reddens further and I think she is going to blow. But she doesn't say much. I'm not sure that she will come back to me to have them redone. It's amazing, but she is more willing to believe what a friend told her about massage than what I told her. And of course she doesn't remember that during our first meeting, I warned her that some patients get capsules.

Patients tend to have extremely selective hearing.

They remember very little of what doctors tell them. One study found that on average they take in about 20 percent of what they hear—and it's almost never about pain, potential complications, or other hazardous side effects. That's why I tend to repeat information in consultations and to put it again on paper. I know it's hard to take it all in at once, but it's important. Now Jolinda is living with this nasty surprise, and she thinks it is due to my failure to encourage massage.

She meets with Lorraine afterward about the price of additional surgery—I will waive my fee, of course, but she will have to pay for the anesthesiologist. But she doesn't set a date to do it, and Lorraine is pretty convinced that she will find a different doctor.

3:30 P.M.

This is my second session with Annabel, a small blond woman who has lost more than a hundred pounds after gastric bypass surgery. In a week, she is going to have her face lifted, tummy tucked, and breasts lifted and enlarged. The surgery will take about five hours, and it has to be done in the hospital because of the length of time she will be under anesthesia. Six months later, when she is all healed, I will fix her arms and thighs.

Annabel found me through a support group where she met another patient who'd undergone the same procedures. Since losing the weight, she looks so drastically different, she says, that at a party her husband said to a group of people, "Let me introduce you to my second wife." And they believed it.

She is excited about the surgery and shows absolutely no concern or fear about what she is facing—at least a week of painful recuperation, mainly from the tummy tuck. I guess she isn't intimidated because she already suffered with her weight all of those years, and the gastric bypass was a far riskier enterprise than the cosmetic work she is contemplating. Her husband is the one with the detailed questions about what she will need and what risks she might face. But he, too, is obviously thrilled that she will be heading into her final transformation.

"When the surgery is over," I tell him, "you can introduce her as your third wife."

3:50 P.M.

After finishing with Annabel, I go into the kitchen. I overhear Lorraine on the telephone with a patient who has called to say she is pregnant. With many patients, we don't become social friends, but we become what I consider personal acquaintances. This patient is worried about her breast implants and whether they will be affected by pregnancy. Having had implants, Lorraine knows how important they become to self-image.

"Don't you worry about those puppies," she tells her. "If there's any problem at all, he'll fix them."

We joke around with the patients, we flirt, we connect. Sometimes, patients talk about very personal things, about their marriages, their sex lives. One of the nice perks of my job is I get lots of presents from patients who are grateful. Today, one of my regular Botox patients gives me one of those little sand gardens with the pebbles and the rakes. Good to know she is happy with her wrinkle-free brow.

My staff member who handles queries from the outside world—

which means marketing, questions from reporters, and issues relating to professional meetings, and journals—comes into the kitchen wanting to know whether I will give a presentation at a meeting coming up in Boston. I'm on the faculty at New York University, and so I teach an occasional seminar. More important, each time I do a procedure at the hospital, there is a fellow or resident in the room with me, and I show him or her how to do surgery. I like narrating what I do and having someone watching, giving me his or her attention. It's fun. I also do a fair amount of paper writing and presenting for professional medical journals and conferences. I usually do the writing late at night, always at the office. I don't like to work at home. After everyone has left the office, I'll start writing and stay until three in the morning if I have to. The most recent one I did had the catchy title of "A Randomized, Double-Blind, Multicenter Comparison of the Efficacy and Tolerability of Restylane Versus Zyplast for the Correction of Nasolabial Folds," published in a journal called *Dermatological Surgery*. Presentations for professional meetings are a little simpler to put together. I recently gave one in New York on the long-term results of forehead lifting, at the Aging Face Symposium.

Lorraine likes to joke that my idea of relaxing is to come into the office on a Sunday and write a paper.

4:10 P.M.

When women come to me for consultations—and most of my patients are women—I always start by asking what they are concerned with, to take a mirror and tell me what bothers them. My job is to look at them and tell them whether I see what they see.

These days, many women are coming in for Restylane injections. Now Marianna is waiting for me in Room 1. She is frustrated with the lines that run from the nose to the mouth, called the nasolabial folds. She is only in her early thirties, but she does have unusually deep lines. I tell her that Restylane is a product newly approved by the FDA and that it has been used in Europe and Canada for a very long time. And that because it is a sugar derivative, it doesn't require any testing ahead of time to check for allergic reactions.

"I hardly ever use collagen anymore, because I don't think it makes sense," I explain. "In addition, Restylane lasts longer."

I then explain that I will give her a shot to numb the area around her gums, just like the dentist does, which will minimize any pain from the injections. Before I do that, I have something that numbs the gum to make the injection easier to take.

"The flavor is piña colada. This takes the edge off."

After I do that, I use a marking pen to draw the places on her face where I will inject the Restylane. When I am sure she is numb, I begin injecting the lines with a series of shots about a tenth of an inch apart until I finish both lines. She is a little red, and her skin is a little swollen, but that is a perfectly normal response. I tell her that her skin will look fine by the next day and that she will see a noticeable difference in the lines within a week or so.

4:30 P.M.

Judith is in her early forties, nice looking in a generic Upper East Side sort of way, with blunt-cut dirty blond hair, a pleasant face and trim body, and understated clothes and shoes. She has been here for three or four sessions to get Botox, and every time she talks about whether she should have a face-lift and what the effects would be.

Today, however, she is obsessed with her thighs. I try to tell her that thigh-lifts are quite unsuccessful because they leave horrible scars, that she really should just go to the gym or work out with a personal trainer, and do what she can do to improve her muscle tone. If she wants surgery, she should focus on her eyes and her face, because that's what people see, and that's also what makes the biggest difference with the least amount of scarring. But I guess she isn't ready to hear that.

Judith is one of my more unusual patients. Women don't usually procrastinate for two years while they come to me for injections. There's some roadblock here. It's not her husband. He is with her this time and talks about having his eyes done. Even though she's never had surgery, she's a good patient. She has sent dozens of people in for surgery, just based on her experience with Botox.

Perhaps next time she'll be ready to take the plunge.

4:45 P.M.

When I get back to the kitchen, Lorraine tells me that I have two more patients backed up in the waiting room. I know people hate to wait, but even more than that, they hate to have doctors rush through consultations and give the impression they don't want to answer questions. And that's what you have to do to run always on time, day in and day out.

So I don't. I think it's worth the trade-off. I like going into great detail with patients about the surgery and what to expect afterward. I think you have to. People are very well educated now, and they have reasonable questions. They go on the Internet. They know about the different incisions. They watch surgery on television, on shows like *Extreme Makeover* or *Nip/Tuck*.

And they talk to their friends.

When I talk about the pros and cons of putting breast implants under the muscle or above the muscle, they usually know what I'm talking about. In the end, an informed patient makes everything easier, for me and for her. It's always better to understand why and how a procedure is done, and the logic behind my decisions. When I go to a doctor's office, I don't want to be informed imperiously that "this is what I'm doing, and that's all I have to say about it." I want to know what's going to happen every step of the way, and I always assume my patients do too.

Unless they inform me otherwise.

It's important, though, to make my patients happy, because they can and will go plastic surgeon shopping. Every time Lorraine goes to another doctor's office for an appointment, she comes back and changes something about our office. She sees the kinds of things that bother her finely honed instincts, and she will not allow them to exist in our office. Things like dirty or smelly bathrooms, or torn carpets, or receptionists eating their lunch or reading the *Star* while they're greeting patients.

Or, worst in her mind, having personal conversations within earshot of the patients in the waiting room.

4:50 P.M.

Jeremiah is next. He's very established in his profession as well as very wealthy as a result, and he wants to talk about having a face-lift. He was referred to me by his internist and says he had no reason not to trust me, but he wants to hire another surgeon, too, and have him watch the surgery to make sure that nothing goes wrong.

"Money is no object," he says. "I just want to make sure I get the best."

I tell him that it is an interesting idea and that in theory I have no objection to it. I often scrub in with my colleagues at the hospital.

"I work with fellows and residents all the time," I say. "But let's say we come to a situation where I want to go right and he or she wants to go left. Do we leave the operating room and go have a cup of coffee and talk about it?"

He likes that answer.

"You're right. I don't need another doctor. You've given me all the confidence I need."

5:15 P.M.

Georgia is at the other extreme from the fastidious and impeccably dressed Jeremiah. She has pulled her long hair back in a ponytail and is clad in scuffed Birkenstock sandals and baggy socks, a purple T-shirt, and well-worn jeans. She doesn't look like she can easily afford surgery.

But appearances can always be deceiving. She may be savvy enough to have dressed down for our meeting. And she is very well informed and full of questions. She wants her nose changed, and she also wants to talk about whether her lips can be made fuller. She is curious too about whether a brow-lift is a possibility. She'd even brought computer print-outs of noses she likes and noses she doesn't.

"I don't like the typical American nose," she says. "The thin nose, the button nose. You know, the perky Meg Ryan nose."

I tell her that people are much less rigid about features these days, and the standard one nose fits all is no longer being done, at least not in New York by anybody competent. I answer all of her questions, but when she leaves, I have no inkling whether I will ever see her again.

5:35 P.M.

At the end of the day, the office staff leaves, and it's just Lorraine and me. I loosen my tie, sit down at my desk, and go over all of the charts of the day, writing the longer notes I didn't have time to make earlier. I answer calls from other doctors, from colleagues with questions, from my attorney, from friends. We're going out to dinner later, and to a concert, so Lorraine slips out to see the kids.

I like putzing around in the now-hushed office. This is my quiet time, my time to wrap everything up.

7 P.M.

I leave the office. I'm always the first to arrive and the last to go. Walking down Park Avenue, I pass the office of my estimable colleagues, Daniel Baker and Sherrell Aston, who are considered among the best doctors in New York and are my colleagues at Manhattan Eye and Ear. Practices differ from surgeon to surgeon. Botox and Restylane injections have become a big part of mine, but not every plastic surgeon does them.

True, it's not the same as doing surgery. But it's a moneymaker, so it's a good thing to have in an office. It also happens to lead to surgery. And, more important in my mind, it builds a long-term relationship. Every time I see a patient, even for a minor treatment for a zit or a wrinkle, I consider that the best public relations I have. I'm not the world's most brilliant conversationalist, but I think that overall I'm a likable person, and I'm presentable, and most of the time I know what I'm talking about. So the individual exposure sells the patients.

Of course, there will always be patients who walk in and talk to me for fifteen minutes and realize they can't stand my guts. I will never have a relationship with them, and I'm willing to accept that. It's just one of those things—you either click and have chemistry, or you don't. But I think that on average patients tend to like me. Exposure counts. If I have fifteen or twenty minutes with a person, and that person likes the way we interact, she might come back in ten years.

And refer her friends.

As much as I love my life, I know that someday I'll have to walk away from my job. This isn't a line of work for old men. You need young, strong eyes and a steady hand. I figure I have another ten, fifteen years before I'm too old to be a top surgeon. And I don't want to do it if I'm not one of the best.

To tell the truth, if I didn't need the money, I'd think about leaving it all and opening an art gallery devoted to the Dadaists I love. But even as I say that, I'm not sure I totally believe it. I had fun today.

I know I'll have fun tomorrow too.

7:20 P.M.

I'm starving. I go east from Park Avenue, over to Lexington Avenue and into Orsay. To me, this place is like an extension of my home. Lorraine is waiting for me when I get there. I've barely said hello before the bartender hands me my usual vodka martini—made with Polish vodka in honor of my homeland—with two olives. We always sit at the same table, where we can look out the window, and I nearly always have steak or fish. We often run into one or more of our patients here, some of whom have no interest whatsoever in acknowledging my existence, which is certainly their prerogative. But it's a slow night. We enjoy our meal, talking about our day, and leave for the concert.

9 P.M.

We take a cab to the Beacon Theater, where the Allman Brothers are playing. Gregg's wife Stacy always calls when they are coming to town and tells us where to meet them. Happily feeling like groupies, we go through the backstage entrance and up to Gregg's dressing room. We hang out while the opening band is playing and talk about what we missed since we last saw one another, about our shared love of political debate and old Harley-Davidsons. Lorraine is starting to nod off at this point, but I'm just getting going. We sit on the stage during the concert, which is such a kick for me. I used to listen to the Allman Brothers when I was a teenager, and sometimes I still can't believe I'm up here.

11:30 P.M.

Home to bed. Lorraine collapses almost immediately. I catch the end of *Nightline,* check all the thermostats in the house to make sure the heat's not too high, make sure the roof door is locked, and then, an hour after arriving home, make my way to bed.

What a great day.

Give this up? I don't know how.

Two

TEN MYTHS ABOUT PLASTIC SURGERY

SOME PEOPLE BELIEVE THAT IF THEY DON'T SMILE, THEY WON'T HAVE smile lines, but that's just ridiculous. There are only two things you can do to make a difference in your skin: protect it from the sun, and do not smoke.

Otherwise, hope for good genes.

Much of the aging process is genetically determined. Inherited problems are unfortunate, and no amount of expensive skin care products can undo them. Save your money for something that will work—like surgery.

If your flaws bug you, and you do decide to have surgery, nothing is more important than finding a qualified, careful surgeon. It's your face, or your body, and once you're on the table in the OR, there's no going back.

Here are ten of the most enduring myths about plastic surgery.

Myth #1: I'll Look Like Joan Rivers

No, you won't. Not unless that's what you want.

On the other hand, right after surgery you may well look like the

Bride of Godzilla, but after the stitches come out and the swelling sub-sides, you'll look a whole lot better. After a face-lift, I tell all my Jewish patients to pretend they're sitting shiva for seven days. Cover the mirrors. It won't do you any good to look in them.

Myth #2: Plastic Surgery Is Painless

There's a reason people take painkillers. They kill the pain.

Plastic surgery can hurt. A little or a lot. Whether by scalpel or laser, if there's no pain, there's no gain.

The amount of pain, however, varies with each procedure and with each patient. Women seem to tolerate pain better than men, but even among women, there is a huge range of reactions to pain. For some, it's merely a matter of discomfort. For many, a face-lift hurts far less than expected—but it may be the worst-*looking* procedure imaginable, espe-cially if it includes laser. Patients are so bloodied and beat up that it hurts their friends and family to look at them, but it doesn't feel as awful as it looks.

Be warned. These are the most painful procedures:

Abdominoplasty, or Tummy Tuck

The surgery can take up to three hours. Medically it's the highest risk of all the procedures I do, because the incision is so large and so much is done with the muscles. This results in significant trauma to the tissue. You'll be immobile for only a day or two, usually moaning in agony if you refuse to take painkillers, and it takes about a month to be fully active again.

Breast Augmentation, or Implants

These can be painful because the implants are put under the muscle, which means the muscle must be cut.

Full-Face Laser

A laser is a burn, and the one used to get rid of facial wrinkles and scars causes a second-degree burn. Ouch. Never trust any doctor who says a laser resurfacing treatment is going to be pain-free. He or she is lying.

Thigh-Lift

The incisions are in the groin area, which is sensitive. Sitting down puts pressure on it. For about two weeks, you can't sit comfortably.

Body-Lift

This is designed for people who've lost significant amounts of weight and have excess, hanging skin. It's an aggressive procedure in which an incision is made all the way around the body. It requires eight hours of general anesthesia and entails blood loss and transfusions. I no longer do it because it isn't worth putting patients through an operation that creates that much stress on the body, with unsatisfactory gains due to large scars.

Myth #3: Plastic Surgery Is Risk Free

If a doctor ever tells you that plastic surgery is risk free, run out the door. Among the risks are hematoma, which is a pooling of blood under the skin; infection, which can be very serious; anesthesia, which can cause severe problems; and permanent nerve injury.

And, of course, death.

Although death from plastic surgery is rare, it is still a risk. Novelist Olivia Goldsmith, who wrote *The First Wives Club*, died in January 2004, during an operation to tighten the skin under her chin. After the anesthesia was administered, her heart stopped; it could have been from a pulmonary embolism or from a heart attack. Maybe the anesthesia was administered incorrectly, or maybe she failed to give the doctor some crucial information. I don't know. But whatever happened, it should reinforce the idea that to reduce risk, it's important to learn everything you can about who will be working on you during surgery and to disclose all pertinent information to your doctor. It's worth a higher fee for a competent, board-certified surgeon and a board-certified anesthesiologist.

Myth #4: Plastic Surgery Lasts Forever

If you want forever, get a diamond.

The minute I close the incision, gravity and the inevitable aging process start their inexorable march. I may have taken ten years off your face, but ten years from now, you'll still look older. You just won't look as old as you would have without the procedure.

For some people, a face-lift lasts for ten or fifteen years. Others are back after seven years. It's a very personal thing.

It's the same with injectibles. In some people, wrinkles injected with a filler stay smooth for a year. Others need another application after six months.

Unfortunately, there's no fail-safe method of predicting how you'll do. Be realistic with your expectations, and you're less likely to be disappointed.

Myth #5: Your Doctor Operates on You and Takes Care of You Afterward

Not always. Some of America's top surgeons routinely meet with their patients for consultations but leave some of the surgical work to assistants. The surgeon makes the incisions but has the resident or fellow sew them up later. That way, a surgeon can have two operating rooms going at once.

Two rooms going at once equals twice as much money.

I never do that. The sewing decides much of the look of the scar. A patient doesn't see what I do under the skin. But that work is vital, because scars are what you see.

Not surprisingly, that kind of volume surgery is difficult to carry out in hospitals. Hospitals don't like it. It gives them added liability. But now that doctors do so much of their surgery in their private operating rooms attached to their offices, it's hard to know exactly what goes on.

Some surgeons also leave most or all of the surgical aftercare, especially on weekends, to the nurses in their offices, or to the residents or fellows. They don't change the dressings or take out the sutures. I also like to do that myself, because that's where problems can be caught early—and cured. If those jobs are left to someone who isn't a doctor, that opportunity may be lost.

So if your surgeon is not totally hands-on after surgery, never schedule your operation for a Friday. And especially not a Friday in the summer, when weekend getaways are a must for doctors—and hell for patients.

When I was younger, I was often the weekend and holiday backup doctor for several prominent surgeons in New York. I am indebted to them, because that helped me build my practice. But for their patients, that meant a disorienting sense of being abandoned if something went wrong. One December, a patient came to see me who'd had a full-face laser treatment to remove bad acne scars. It's serious business. Lasers burn skin, leaving it weepy and red. Patients need to hide out at home for a week afterward. She came to see me because she was worried that she wasn't healing correctly, and she was right. There were some areas that looked like bad, still-open scrapes. Although they were only superficial abrasions, she should have been in better shape at that point. I thought she might have an infection, so I put her on antifungal drugs and oral antibiotics, and I took some cultures so the lab could figure out what was going on. I told her to call me the next day if she wasn't better.

She did. It was New Year's Eve—I remember, because it was the only time I ever met with a patient wearing my tuxedo. I was horrified. She had a massive infection. Her skin had started to melt away in patches. It scared the living daylights out of me. I had her rushed to the hospital and put on intravenous antibiotics. It turned out to be an infection caused by an uncommon organism usually found in the intestinal tract. The only thing I could figure was that she had touched something that someone else with inappropriate hygiene had touched, and then touched her face. She was in the hospital for five days. The infection healed, but of course she still had to heal at home from the laser. She recovered and luckily ended up with only superficial scarring. She was so grateful that I had taken care of her when her surgeon had been out of town, that she came to me for cheek implants three years later.

Myth #6: You Can Get a Nose Job on Your Lunch Hour

There are doctors who advertise "lunch hour" surgical procedures. Even if people don't literally want to go back to work after the procedures, they are attracted by the idea that their recovery is going to be quick.

Then they find out the real meaning of "quick." It's not a lunch hour. It's a lot longer.

These procedures might sound minor, especially when promoted as simpler and faster, but once an incision is made, it's there forever. It's not always possible to fix it.

There was a doctor who promised patients he could remake their noses during a lunch hour. Indeed he did. He would numb the nose and then shave the dorsal bone. The usual procedure is to break the bone and then refashion it. Well, guess what the patients needed after he finished? The rest of the rhinoplasty.

This doctor left the nose open at the top. Touching it would create a small depression because the bones were no longer meeting. I had to do the second part of the procedure for these patients. And none of them was happy about it.

Myth #7: Silicone Implants Are Better Than Saline

Years ago, that was true. Silicone gel was better because it was softer. The older saline implants, which were silicone bags filled with salt water, had thick shells and a lot of ridging, and you could feel everything. That made for a very awkward bag of salt water.

Now the bags are thinner and of much higher quality. There is no reason to get silicone except for a breast reconstruction after a mastectomy. I can guarantee that if I gave you a silicone implant in one breast and a saline implant in the other, you wouldn't be able to tell the difference.

Myth #8: Some Surgeons Can Deliver Scarless Surgery

No way. We've grown much more sophisticated about concealing scars in natural creases of the body, but they're still there. Any doctor who says he or she can do a scarless procedure is not telling the truth. A breast-lift or a face-lift can be scarless only if there are no incisions . . . and if there are no incisions, it's not surgery. It's a con.

Myth #9: If I Saw It on TV, It Must Be True

Maybe if you're watching TV in some other universe. Many surgeons hire savvy public relations companies to create savvy public relations campaigns for them. Viewers are interested in health and beauty, and more viewers results in more advertising revenue. Some sexy young hot-shot surgeon claiming to be the "only one" to have a unique technique honed at the feet of Ponce de León is going to get air time. Is this hot shot any good? Maybe. Is his PR effective? Undoubtedly. That doesn't mean he's the best doctor for you.

Remember that most surgical refinements are carried out by a number of surgeons working all over the world. No one surgeon can take credit for having developed any of the big procedures. And no one surgeon has a monopoly on them. We all have access to pretty much the same tools. Change comes through a steady process as procedures are refined; it's an evolution, not a revolution. With face-lifts, for example, we first concentrated on the importance of the underlying muscle; the next big thing was the placement of scars behind the ears, which made them less visible. More recently, we have been developing advances in how we handle the malar fat pads, which are under the cheeks and, in their proper position, give the face a more youthful look.

Myth #10: New Is Always Better

Better! Faster! Different! Cutting-edge! Bad pun!

Doctors are always sniffing around the brand-new rather than the tried-and-true. Don't fall for the hype.

New techniques and methods are not always better. Sometimes they are worse. Artecoll, which is being touted as a replacement for collagen, is not better. It can leave hard little pellets in the skin. Yet these supposedly new procedures are written about as if they're the best thing ever to have happened. New materials and procedures have to prove themselves over time. This means years, not months. I need proof that they're going to work in the long run.

Take external ultrasonic liposuction. A few years ago we were told that if you took this device and rubbed it on the skin, it would break up fat. Doctors bought the machine because they wanted to be the first ones in their neighborhood to have it.

But it didn't work.

I wasn't snookered by that one, but I did once buy a highly touted device from someone I trusted. It was a suction device based on the idea of stretching and enlarging breast tissue, and my colleague said it would help enlarge breasts for patients who couldn't have surgery because breast cancer ran in their families. I used it on three patients. All three had allergic reactions.

That device was the hot new thing. For about five hot minutes.

Three

NUTS FOR NEEDLES: BOTOX AND BEYOND

ONE OF MY PATIENTS WAS IN A CAR ACCIDENT. WHEN SHE GOT TO THE hospital, the admitting doctor examined her for neurological damage. He asked her to look to the left, to the right, and then up. When she looked up but her forehead didn't budge, he became concerned.

"Wrinkle your forehead," he said.

"Are you kidding?" she replied. "I can't raise my brows. My Botox cost a fortune!"

The American Society for Aesthetic Plastic Surgery estimates that 2.3 million injections of Botox were given in 2003, and that number is growing. Ever since it was approved by the FDA in 2001 for cosmetic use, Botox, the product name for a purified and diluted form of the nontoxic botulinum toxin type A, which paralyses the muscles that cause wrinkles, has become the most popular cosmetic procedure in America. Take a look at your favorite celebrities, and you'll see why. Smooth, unwrinkled brows are no longer a mirage. Botox has made it possible to nearly eliminate lines on the forehead, between the eyebrows, and to a lesser extent, around the eyes.

Botox is only one of what we call "injectibles." Unlike Botox, most injectibles act as fillers—substances that plump up the area around lines, filling them in. They can help postpone the need for surgery, or avoid it altogether. The correction they provide is not as significant as surgery, but the process is also not as painful, time-consuming—or expensive.

Injecting Botox is not difficult, but it's what we refer to as a "technique-dependent therapy." This means that an inexperienced doctor applying Botox can mess up your face. It won't lead to any permanent distortion, because the substance wears off after six or seven months, but injectibles are not as easy as they look. An intimate knowledge of anatomy is a pre-requisite.

Because patients have heard some scary stories about Botox parties, and about faces that have become totally expressionless or eyebrows that droop, some of them are very nervous when they first come in for the shots. For everyone, the process is the same. I look for problem creases, figure out where and how Botox can help, and educate them about the substance.

"Raise your eyebrows, please, and look really, really angry," I said to a new patient, a thirty-eight-year-old lawyer from Connecticut named Kelly.

Kelly scowled, revealing all of the creases in her forehead. With an erasable-ink pen, I highlighted all the lines I would soon inject with Botox.

"Now squint," I said and proceeded to mark the lines around her eyes.

"I played a lot of tennis growing up, and I guess I squinted into the sun too much," she said sheepishly.

Patients like Kelly—well educated and successful in intellectual professions—often feel they have to give an excuse for having landed in my office. I try to ease away their self-consciousness.

"I get Botox too," I said. "My twin brother is a dermatologist in California, and he does it for me. So I know what it's like."

What it's like is painful. But the pain doesn't last long, and the results can be stunning.

"The only thing I don't want is flat eyebrows," Kelly said. Having read many magazine articles about Botox, she knew that if it was injected too far to the right of the center of the eyebrow, the eyebrow would droop. But that's not a consequence of Botox—it's a mistake by a doctor who injected into the wrong place.

"Don't worry, I always stop at the midpupillary line," I told her. "I know what you mean, though. If you inject incorrectly, you drop the brow and get a very bland expression."

I asked if she had any medical problems or allergies to penicillin or codeine. It's a routine question, but in fact there is no need to pretest for Botox, because it does not produce allergic reactions. I ask these questions as part of a patient's medical history, in case it becomes relevant. "Botox's results can last anywhere from three to six months," I said. "The results aren't immediately obvious, which is sometimes frustrating to first-time users. It takes about two days to see a difference. Sometimes, there is a bit of bruising after the injections."

She nodded.

"Don't exercise today," I went on. It wouldn't hurt her, but it could lead to a bit of swelling in the forehead if she did anything that involved straining, like weight lifting, or bending over, like vigorous aerobics.

"I already worked out."

"Great. Now here are the risks." I tell every new patient about possible risks, no matter how remote. "If I inject below the orbital rim, I can inactivate the muscle that elevates the eyelid," I explained as I wiped her forehead with EMLA, a topical anesthetic cream that dulls the pain a bit. "It's unlikely. These are technical errors. Botox doesn't travel."

"Fine. I'm all ready."

I picked up the phone and asked one of my assistants to bring in a waiver. Before any injection or surgery or procedure, patients must sign documents saying that they understand what they are getting and the risks and benefits. It's mandatory for insurance companies, in case of potential lawsuits.

"Here we go." I wiped off the EMLA and began injecting. I try to keep conversations going whenever patients seem to want to talk. It distracts them and makes it easier to bear the pain. "I just discovered something very interesting," I told her. "I did a brow-lift for a symposium on a patient who has been coming to me for three years for regular Botox. I noticed this muscle in her was almost completely gone. There'd been suggestions that the Botox permanently deactivates the muscle, but I never believed it. Until I saw that."

Kelly didn't care about muscles. She was wincing and grimacing, and finally said the needles hurt terribly, even with the EMLA.

"Try to relax. I'm nearly done."

"Plus I'm scared because I haven't done it before," she admitted.

I finished her brow lines, and suggested we take a breather so she could be ready for the next assault.

"You should see me when I get Botox," I said. "I can sympathize with what you're going through."

She managed a weak smile as I started injecting around her eyes.

"In this location, believe it or not, it's less painful." After each injection, I put a little pressure against the skin to minimize any black-and-blue marks. "If you're going to bruise, it happens now. It means you're bleeding a little. That's all."

I pointed out a patent that I'd framed and hung on the wall next to her chair. It was for a device I developed in the course of creating techniques for the endoscopic brow-lift, which returns the forehead to its original position through a surgery that requires fewer incisions than the previous method.

"You'll like this story," I said, "because you're a lawyer. This company sent me an e-mail saying they'd devised an absorbable suspension device and would like me to use it. I told them to bring it in. Their rep came and showed me a device similar to what I'd patented in 1997. I told him I'd think about it—and then I called my attorney."

"It happens all the time," she said.

She seemed a little less tense, but this clearly was torture. She kept making little sighing noises, trying to get through the pain. It's funny with Botox. Some people don't make a sound, and they're so relaxed you'd think they were sitting on the beach downing margaritas. Others are in agony.

"You're almost there," I said, wondering if she'd be back. Unlikely, unless the results were so appealing that she decided the pain was worth it.

Botox has completely changed the business of plastic surgery, bringing in patients who would never consider going under the knife. Once they get accustomed to being worked on, though, they often change their minds.

"Okay," I told Kelly. "You survived."

She visibly relaxed.

"Use this ice pack. You can reuse it—just pop it in the freezer. Tonight, you can use makeup if you wish."

After Kelly left, I went to the kitchen and filled out her chart. It makes me nuts, all this paperwork. I can't delegate it. Just as I finished grumbling, Alan, our Botox salesman, arrived with some new videos we can show to our patients at the auxiliary practice I'm setting up at a spa and hospital in Montego Bay, Jamaica. I told him about the disappearing muscles I'd discovered the other day during the endoscopic brow-lift.

"So the atrophy effect is real," he said.

"I never really believed that," I said.

"We've theorized it, but it would be interesting to develop some proof."

"Well, I have proof. And it's on videotape."

"So we don't paralyze. We eliminate," Alan said. "I always say it's the opposite of exercise. We atrophy the muscle. This means we can start researching Botox use in younger people, to see whether it works as a prophylactic, as a way to prevent wrinkles. That would be awesome."

The applications are expanding. If applied judiciously Botox can even be used around the mouth. It can sometimes be used, too, on the neck, in the platysma band, the muscles directly below the chin that in some people are very pronounced.

Lunch arrived, and Lorraine asked me if I had any money to pay the delivery person.

"I have exactly one dollar in my pocket," I retorted. "I see patients, I eat what's put in front of me, then I go back and see more patients."

Lorraine stuck out her tongue and went to pay. Alan turned on the video.

"The first thing people want to know about is safety," he said. "We think it's important to tell them that Botox has been used therapeutically for ten years, to make them feel more confident that they're not guinea pigs for some cosmetic treatment."

Botox was used for years off-label, meaning it hadn't been specifically approved for cosmetic purposes, but it had been tested and approved for other uses that involved paralyzing muscles—for blepharospasm, when the muscle around the eye is continually going into spasms, and for Parkinson's, to relax the muscle rigidity that affects people with that disease. When the FDA did give it the go-ahead in 2001 for cosmetic applications, it was actually approved only for the frown lines that develop between the eyebrows, called glabellar lines. Technically, all other uses, including for forehead creases, are not officially approved by the FDA.

As if anybody cares.

"What about the doses?" I asked. Although doctors may talk to other doctors at symposia, in daily business, drug reps like Alan are the only ones who know what the doctors up the street are really doing.

And when the street is Park Avenue, that means a lot of doctors are breathing down each other's necks.

"The range is all over the block," he said. "Between seven and fifteen units per side on the crow's-feet. On the forehead, it's between twenty and forty units in females. Males are forty to sixty. But plenty of guys are getting effective results with less, using from fifteen to twenty to fifty units. The shapes and lines are different on everybody, and you can't tell by the depth of the lines."

"I use about twenty-five units on female foreheads. Men do tend to need much more."

Because it is impossible to know exactly how much Botox a patient needs to get optimum results, Alan recommended starting low and then adding more if the result wasn't good enough. At least that offers a baseline. Then he added that the median price for a treatment in the

Park Avenue neighborhood was $1,200, but some doctors were charging only $450.

I found that low price hard to believe. They'd be administering Botox at cost, which made no sense. "Are they diluting the doses?" I asked.

"No way," he replied. "We've watched it done. They're not."

I just didn't think that was possible, unless some doctors were using it as a lure to bring in patients who might move on to other treatments. Not that Botox couldn't be found in plenty of places for less than I charge. Doctors who offer Botox at bargain-basement prices put much less in the syringe. There's nothing wrong with that, but patients should understand that a small amount of Botox won't last five or six months; it will last one or two. Users usually chalk up the disappointing results to Botox, without realizing that they didn't receive optimal amounts.

Alan left for his next appointment, and I went to see my next patient. Waiting, of course, for Botox. It was one of my regulars, Joanna, who was in her early fifties.

"How are you?" I asked. "I haven't seen you in a while."

"I went to the south of France for the summer."

"Lucky you," I said, looking at her forehead. "Pretend you're really angry at me."

She knew the drill. I could see that most of the effects of her last treatment had worn off. She told me she particularly wanted me to pay attention to the left side, that it had returned to normal faster than the other side. That was the variability that Alan talked about. You don't know how much Botox you need in a particular spot except by trial and error.

"My daughter came to see you for Restylane," she said. "It left a bump on the side of her lip."

"Really?" I was surprised. Restylane is a filler that goes around the mouth area. "I might be able to inject on the other side. Tell her to come in and I'll take care of it."

It's not unusual for me to treat several members of one family. In one case, I did a face-lift on the grandmother, a breast implant on the mother, and a rhinoplasty on the teenage daughter.

I asked Joanna to scrunch up her face again so I could mark the sites for the injections. As I put on my loupes—supermagnifying glasses that make me look like a giant bug—and went about my work, the room fell silent. Joanna was so relaxed she didn't even flinch at the injections.

"You're a great patient," I said. "I should videotape you and advertise you as my poster child for Botox."

She smiled but otherwise didn't make a move. All you could hear was the sound of the needle puncturing her skin.

In another minute, she was finished. I handed her an ice pack, told her to sit with it for a half hour in the waiting room, and to ice as much as she could when she got home, to cut down on bruising.

Then I went to see my next patient, Joanna's cousin, forty-eight-year-old Lois.

"Your cousin is amazing," I told Lois. "It's so easy to give her the injections. But you're pretty stoic too."

Lois laughed. She was a bleeder and tends to get much more black and blue.

Not that it would stop her from coming back for more.

So enough already about Botox. Newer injectibles that can be used to fill in lines around the nose and mouth are becoming increasingly popular. For a number of years, collagen had been the drug of choice. But now I believe Restylane will soon replace collagen. I'm a big fan. It lasts longer, and unlike collagen, it's not made from any human or animal products. And because it's a sugar molecule, hyaluronic acid, it can't provoke an allergic reaction, so it doesn't require allergy testing. I was part of the Restylane study mandated by the FDA as part of the approval process, sponsored by Q-Med, the Swedish company that developed it. Because of my experience, I have been asked to become a member of the medical advisory board for Restylane's distributor.

Another injectible alternative is Hylaform. Recently approved by the FDA, this form of hyaluronic acid is derived from rooster combs.

Other products have less appeal, and I'm reluctant to use them. Artecoll, made from tiny plastic polymeric microspheres placed in collagen, is supposed to fill wrinkles permanently. I don't like it because if the result isn't perfect, the problems are also permanent. After the collagen is absorbed by the body, the tiny plastic spheres remain and can leave ugly lumps.

Frankly, any injectible that can be permanent concerns me. People are especially eager to try out injectibles because they think they're safer than surgery. So they run out and get silicone injections to plump up lips and cheeks, and there are some awful consequences that I am called upon to fix. Silicone can migrate, leaving lumpy skin. It can cause skin eruptions too. Plus lips can be made overly large, disproportionate to the face, and sometimes permanently so. Sometimes I can cut some of it out, but lips will never get back to normal.

Although the risk with a temporary injectible is not as great, none comes with any guarantees. For one thing, everybody processes these substances differently. For another, which is even more important, putting things in the face is never simple. Some problems arise because people are obsessed with the newest treatments or substances. They read one article in a magazine or find some site on the Internet, and are convinced this is the ticket back to their youth. They don't understand that just because something's been praised in print doesn't mean it actually works.

Take Gore-Tex, a synthetic material chemically called polytetrafluoroethylene that can be implanted in parts of the body—in some cases, to great advantage. But not always. One of the worst things you can do is get Gore-Tex or SoftForm (another name for Gore-Tex) implants in your lips. It never makes sense to put a rigid substance like Gore-Tex into a dynamic area like the mouth. Every time you smile or pucker up, you'll look like you have a brick in your upper lip.

I sure wouldn't want to kiss that.

Another thing people do to enhance the lip involves surgery, where a strip of skin is removed, and the upper red line is moved up. The incision is placed right along the red line, and the lip is enlarged below it. These scars are horrible. At best, lips look artificial, and they appear funny when you smile and talk. At worst, you can look like you've had a botched repair of a cleft lip. I've corrected a number of these horrible lip jobs, usually on attractive, younger women.

Sometimes patients are harmed by their own naïveté. Other times, their impatience for perfection drives them to ask doctors to do things that shouldn't be done.

Unfortunately, it's always possible to find a doctor happy to give a patient (and his or her bank account) short-term satisfaction without worrying about the long-term results. Recently, for example, I saw a patient who'd had Kenalog, which is a long-acting steroid, injected into a scar after surgery, to soften it. That's a big mistake. If you inject Kenalog before the scar has naturally softened, you'll end up with a depression. The skin can look papery and thinned out, and sometimes tiny, new unattractive blood vessels form. I see this all the time. There's no reason whatsoever to do this.

Except greed.

Other patients have unreasonable expectations. One of them, thirty-six-year-old Elaine, was waiting for me. She'd come for Restylane as part of the study I'd done and had been thrilled with the results. About six months later, she came back for more. This time, she wasn't so happy with the results. Two weeks after the injection, she called, complaining that she didn't see much change in her face.

Lorraine had told her that perhaps she should have had more than one syringe, and it was a mistake to expect one dose to take care of all the changes she envisioned, but that if she'd come back, we'd take another look and try to correct what was making her unhappy. This is annoying, but it's still smart business. If Elaine becomes a regular patient, we might have a relationship that lasts until my retirement.

But I had a sneaking suspicion there was a simple reason for Elaine's unhappiness: the cost. Each treatment costs $850. I had no idea whether Elaine could afford it, as she hadn't filled in the line about her employment on her patient information sheet. Many of my patients deliberately leave that line blank. Frankly, I couldn't care less what they do. Stripper or schoolteacher, they're all treated the same.

Now Elaine looked pissed. "When I saw my sister the other day," she said, "she told me that I didn't look any different and had wasted my money. I was really upset because I had just gotten the injection."

There *was* a difference, but Elaine wanted a total elimination of the nasolabial fold. I told her that people get more of a change than they realize, but because no one really remembers (or *wants* to remember) exactly how she looked before the procedure, she underestimates the improvement. Some patients come back complaining that their face-lift didn't produce much change—until I show them their mandatory pre-op photographs.

That usually does the trick.

For injectibles, however, I don't require pre- and post-op photos. Maybe I should. People are more likely to be disappointed in results, or not to understand exactly what has happened if the changes are subtle. Usually the treatment hasn't failed. What's failed is their ability or desire to remember what they looked like before.

"I just want it flat and smooth," Elaine went on, pressing her face with her hand to eliminate that line. "I have such a long face. After my first injection, my sister said my face didn't look long anymore." Then she opened a copy of *Elle* magazine from the waiting room and pointed to a photo of a model.

"Is there any way that I could ever look like this?" she asked. "See how she has these nice full lips?"

Of course she couldn't look like the model, for several reasons. She wasn't beautiful, and she didn't have a perfect camera-ready body. "This photo is completely air-brushed and computer-enhanced," I said. "I think it is reasonable to put some more in your lips, but no one naturally looks like that."

"I hate feeling like I have little hard bony lips," she said.

"Okay," I said, taking the mirror back and putting it on the counter. "I'll go get the Restylane, and I'll send my assistant in."

I wanted my assistant to talk to her about the cost of this new injection. I didn't want there to be any surprises about the cost. It creates ill will if patients are surprised when they have to pay.

When I returned, Elaine was smiling. She had been told that we'd cut the price of this treatment in half.

"I'm so happy," she said, putting her head back in the chair so that I could give her the pain block and then the shots. While I was waiting for the block to take effect, I marked the lines on her face where I planned to make the injections. Marking is crucial not only in surgery but also in small procedures like this, because once I start working, the skin can become distorted, and that makes it easy to make mistakes.

"Go for it. Give me lots and lots. Pretend I'm Goldie Hawn in *The First Wives Club*," she said.

I laughed.

"Do you think my face is too long?" she asked.

I wanted her to feel better about herself without actually denying the fact that her face was indeed on the long side.

"We're all different. Our anatomies are different. I wouldn't do anything surgically to change the length of your face," I said diplomatically.

"You already told me I could use rhinoplasty," she said.

"We did discuss that, and it's entirely your call. You already had a rhinoplasty as a teenager."

"Bad, right?" she said.

"I didn't say that," I said.

I wanted to get her off the subject of her perceived imperfections, so I started talking about dogs. I knew she had a miniature poodle, and I once had a rottweiler named Spike.

"Did I ever tell you how Spike got his name?" I asked as I started injecting her lips with the numbing medicine. Normally I do this only for the upper lip, as some people freak when their entire mouth is frozen for an hour or so, but Elaine insisted.

"When I was an intern at NYU, there was a cardiac fellow. He was tough as nails," I went on. "When he walked into the room people would shake in their boots, but he was actually very kind. He looked like a spike because his waist was twenty-eight inches and his shoulders were fifty-two inches, and from the back he looked like a rottweiler strutting. And the name Spike suited him."

Elaine wasn't listening. "Make me look good, okay?" she said. "I have this new boyfriend. Well, okay, we've only gone on two dates, so this is the perfect time to do this as I reel him in. Once he gets to know me better, I don't want him to say, 'Wait a minute, your face looks all different.'"

"I understand," I murmured as I began injecting, placing each shot about a tenth of an inch from the one before, working down the line around her mouth and then into her lips.

"Do you think my face should be fuller?" Elaine asked.

I could see that this topic was going to be unavoidable. For some patients, this topic will always be unavoidable.

Even though I thought her face was fine, I told her the options. "Fat injection is one way to make the face fuller, if that's what you want. Usually I do it in the cheeks. It's pretty neat. It usually takes two injections. I inject six weeks apart in order to let the fat cells incorporate."

"Bring it on," she said. I knew she wasn't ready to do that, but if she really did want to change her face, she had options.

I finished the Restylane and told her to be patient, that it would take a few days to see the ultimate result. The substance is hydrophilic, meaning it draws in water, and the plumping-up process can take several days.

Elaine was no longer pissed. In fact, she was gushingly grateful.

"You're welcome. I always urge my patients to come in again if they're not happy. The worst thing is miscommunication."

But as I said already, it wasn't miscommunication. It was calculation. It made more sense to do a procedure essentially for free and keep a patient likely to become a regular than have her be disappointed and go to another doctor. It's part of the consequence of working with new materials. People sometimes have unrealistic expectations, and until they become familiar with what's possible, it's not surprising that there are problems.

On the other hand, some women keep using Restylane and Botox when they would be better off with surgery. They may be scared of the scalpel, or just don't like the idea.

My next patient, Brenda, was like that. In her forties, with long bleached blond hair and an expensive silk shirt, she was very attractive yet showing her age. She'd been thinking about a face-lift, and this was now her fourth appointment for injectibles. We talk each time about surgery, but she's just not ready.

"Are you happy with the results?" I asked.

"Absolutely," she said. "No one wants to grow old."

I agreed wholeheartedly.

"So tell me how a face-lift can help."

I told her, but I knew she'd be back six months later, patiently enduring the injections.

Four

THE LONG ROAD TO PARK AVENUE

I LOVE WHAT I DO, BUT I NEVER EXPECTED TO BE DOING IT. I WANTED TO be a neurosurgeon or a cardiovascular surgeon. They were the important ones, the fearless surgical cowboys everyone looked up to. To me, plastic surgeons weren't "real" surgeons. When I was in medical school, plastic surgeons were almost embarrassed to say what they did for a living. They'd eagerly talk about the facial reconstructions done on car accident victims but were usually reluctant to admit they offered any purely cosmetic procedures, which are, by medical definition, unnecessary. The standard line was that it was okay to play God in certain cases, like cancer, but that helping people feel better by improving their appearance was no more than shameless, selfish, silly vanity.

My father had been a prominent urologist and general surgeon in Poland, and his father had been the chief lawyer for the Austro-Hungarian Empire. On my mother's side we were descended from nobility, and her father owned knitting mills in Poland. I was born, along with my identical twin brother, Marek, on January 14, 1955. I was five minutes older, and I never let him forget it. I grew up with Marek, my two sisters, Dorota and Elizabeth, my parents, and a few servants in a very large four-bedroom apartment in Warsaw. My grandparents had owned the entire building, but when the Communists took over they confiscated it and left the family with just one apartment, and we even had to pay rent. Still, it was equivalent to a posh street on Manhattan's Upper East Side, and compared to most people, we were privileged. We even had a country place.

My brother and I looked so much alike as kids that my mother joked that she'd have to tie a ribbon on the foot of the one she'd already fed so she wouldn't feed him twice. I spent most of my time at home with my mother and sisters and Marek. I didn't see my father very much. He had a government job working in socialized medicine, but on the side he had a private practice, and he worked late at night and on the weekends. Sunday dinner was family time. It was a happy childhood, but very odd, because of the contrast between public and private life. At school—I'll never forget this—I had to make a poster celebrating the Russian Revolution. But it was a system that had taken nearly everything material away from my family, and it even tried to steal the spiritual, although it didn't succeed. We took religious classes, but we had to hide that from our friends, because we were forbidden to practice our religion by the state.

My father was a stern and proud man, and he refused to become a member of the Communist Party. Professionally, he suffered for it, and his advancement was stymied. More important, he soon realized that his children could never have the life he wanted for them in Poland. He and my mother came up with a plan to escape and go to America, but they told us nothing about it, because they were afraid we would let it slip in conversation with our friends. I remember telling everyone when school got out, "See you in September." It was the summer of 1967, and we were told that we would be going on a camping trip to Yugoslavia. Just before we left, my parents had the apartment painted, which was a sure sign to all the neighbors that we would be coming back. We left Poland in two cars, with my uncle driving my sisters and my cousin, and my brother and I with our parents. We drove to the border and crossed in two different places. We met at a campground, and I remember sitting around the campfire in a rainstorm, and my parents telling us that we were going to America. I was very excited, because it seemed like a big adventure. You always heard about America, about big cars and big cities. My sisters were older, and they were very upset. They didn't want to leave their friends.

The next morning my uncle and cousin left to go back to Poland, and the six of us got into this little German car, with just two suitcases and our camping gear. We drove to the Austrian border, where my mother had a cousin. My father parked the car in a cemetery on the Yugoslav side of the border and let the air out of the tires, so if any policemen came along and asked what we were doing he could say the car had broken down. We picked up our suitcases and got ready to walk through the forest to the Austrian side. My father, who had a whole life as a successful doctor in Poland, started to cry and said that he just couldn't do it. My mother pulled at his lapels and told him we were going.

He knew she was right, and at that moment he stopped thinking about the past and began leading us into our future.

We walked a few miles through the forest with my father at the front and my mother at the end. We were almost there, we could see the border, when a guard started running after us from the Yugoslav side. My mother yelled at us to run, and we did, and the guard was shouting, "I'll shoot."

My mother stopped and looked at him and said, "You have to be a human being. You can't shoot us." My mother was incredibly brave. Many of her friends died in the Warsaw uprising and in concentration camps. The guard put down his gun, and she ran to join us.

We were met on the other side by our relatives. The next day, my father went to Vienna and applied for political asylum, and then he went to seek permission to immigrate to the states. It took three months. In October we flew to JFK. They took us to our new school in the United States the very next day.

From those beginnings, I never dreamed I would end up with a practice on Park Avenue.

We started school right away at North Shore Junior High School in

Glen Head, New York, where my cousin Konrad went. After a few months, by watching the news and cartoons, we were fluent in English.

When we had enough money to get our own place, we moved to a house in Sea Cliff, another small town on the north shore of Long Island. My father had become licensed as a general practitioner. He couldn't start over and become certified as an urologist here. Now that I'm older, it amazes me that he gave up the specialty he loved simply for the idea of a future that might be awaiting his children.

It was culture shock at first. You could go to a supermarket and find oranges and bananas. In Poland, everything was rationed. Some things were familiar. We'd watched *Bonanza* and *Mr. Ed* in Poland, so the television was a link.

All of us had jobs on the weekends to make money for the family. In the beginning, we all worked in the knitting factory that was owned by my relatives. My parents were very strict and demanding. I remember one time in the tenth grade, I had my first taste of alcohol with my friends at a party, and when I came home, my father must have seen that I had been drinking, because he told me to go upstairs and read about Napoleon, and then he made me come downstairs and he quizzed me. That sobered me right up.

Now you know why I have such a strict work ethic.

My father was adamant that we tell the truth. When we were kids, just ten or eleven, my father gave us money and our nanny took us to an amusement park. I spent all of my money on candy and rides. But Marek spent only half of his and hid the rest under his pillow. My father found out and was furious, spanking Marek. He obviously didn't mind that he saved money; he was upset that Marek had hidden something from him.

Now you know why I always tell my patients the truth. In a palatable manner, of course, but the truth must be told.

My parents didn't become rich, but they still managed to pay for all of us to be educated. I went to college at the State University of New York at Stony Brook and then to Albany Medical College. My brother went to the same schools. When we were applying to medical school, my father told us whoever got the higher score on the MCATs could have one of his favorite possessions, a sailboat painted by an eighteenth-century Dutch artist. Luckily for him, he got to keep it, as my brother and I both got exactly the same score: 720 out of 800.

After medical school, I did my internship and residency at New York University's program in surgery at Bellevue Hospital in Manhattan, while Marek went to Ohio State to do his residency in dermatology. NYU was known to be the hardest, toughest, most brutal program in the country. It was not for the faint of heart. It was work, work, and more work, with no frills, no respite, and no perks, other than the privilege of training with the best.

My most vivid memory is that the pancakes in the cafeteria were so awful that we'd drown them in fake syrup to make them edible, and they were still better than any of the other slop on the menu. We were too exhausted to care. I was on call every other night. I'd arrive at five-thirty A.M., do surgery all day, then do surgery all night, and then I'd have to stay there the entire next day taking care of patients. We all did. At nine or ten that night, I'd finally leave. I'd go home and pass out. Get up at five A.M. and start all over again.

In those days, all I wanted was to emulate the Texas tough guy cardiac surgeons and be accepted by them. I did the same things they did. I wore cowboy boots. I chased skirts like crazy. I wouldn't call it dating—I didn't have the energy to get serious. If I had a spare moment I went out drinking with my colleagues.

INTRINSIC ASPECTS OF THE SURGEON'S PERSONALITY
1. Needs immediate gratification—not like an internist, who can dither around with something for six months or longer, especially when dealing with long-term illnesses.
2. Thinks in black and white. To surgeons, there's no such thing as gray. That's for the internists and the gynecologists.
3. Can live with consequences. There are consequences as a surgeon, things you just can't take back. Like a patient dying even as you try frantically to save him.

4. Able to compartmentalize. You can't lose your nerve because of life-and-death situations.

5. Comfortable with himself or herself.

6. Understands and learns from a mistake and doesn't dwell on it. In surgery, you can't say, "Just because this breast implant became infected, I'll never do breast implants again." Get up on the OR horse and do it again.

7. Makes instant decisions.

8. Is a benevolent dictator. You're in charge in the OR, but you've still got to be a team player.

9. Desire to play God.

10. A decent sense of humor.

But after a couple of years, the cowboy allure started to wear off. The cardiac surgeons and neurosurgeons had the most psycho personalities of anyone I have ever met. It's not hard to understand why. You're dealing with the ultimate. Patients are desperately ill. They die with their hearts—literally—in your hands. You have to tell their loved ones. Often, you have no time to think, other than to get in there. One night I opened somebody's chest without any gloves on, intent on saving him, with only seconds to do it. I didn't realize I didn't have gloves on until I was finished. My adrenaline was flowing, and then I looked down and thought, Oh, shit. No fucking gloves. And the young man died anyway.

To say that work like that takes a toll is a vast understatement. One time, we were doing a simple mitral valve replacement, and the patient, a woman in her sixties, died on the table. We tried everything, but we couldn't get her heart going, couldn't get her blood pressure up. Once we knew she was gone, the attending surgeon ripped off his gown and started screaming, "Motherfucker, motherfucker!" Then he yanked the aortic balloon pump out of her groin and splattered blood all over the walls in frustration. He screamed and kicked over one of the carts . . . then went to find the family and give them the awful news.

You'd work your own heart out trying to save people, and sometimes your only thanks was your personal satisfaction. I'll never forget a homeless man named Jimmy. We saved his life and babied him through the intensive care unit. A few weeks later, when I was stumbling out of work one morning, beyond exhaustion, I saw him out on the street drinking. He asked me for a dollar. He had no idea that I was one of the residents who'd saved him.

Another time, I fell asleep holding a heart. As a second assistant in the operating room, my task was to stand to the side and hold the heart during surgery. Well, I'd been up for thirty-six hours straight. The next thing I knew, someone was kicking me under the table, because I'd begun dozing standing up.

If your superiors caught you nodding off, you'd get punished for it. One attending surgeon was forever calling me at one in the morning to tell me he wanted to make rounds. He liked to torture his underlings, especially when he was drunk. On rounds, we always started with a patient's temperature and weight. He'd yell, "Stop!" I'd say, "Yes, sir?" He'd say, "I want the *weight* first and the *temperature* second." I'd tell him, and he'd yell, "Stop! I want the *temperature* first and the *weight* second." It was humiliating for me and especially for the patient. But he didn't care. He was the top dog, and everyone had to know it. Plus he knew that we weren't about to go to the head of the department and say, "Dr. Chief Resident Asshole is picking on me." We were so focused on achieving our goals and getting the hell out that we swallowed our dignity and did what we were told.

I had friends whose marriages fell apart. Friends who died. One senior resident made an intern believe that he had killed a patient. He went home that night and hanged himself.

My idea about what I wanted to be began to change in my second year of residency when I took an elective in plastic surgery, focusing on cranial-facial apsects and taught by Dr. Joe McCarthy, a professor at NYU. It was extraordinary—he made me fall in love with plastic surgery. I experienced it with him; I saw the changes he would make in a person's face. I also realized it is the only discipline where you can be an artist. You're literally resculpting faces and bodies. After I finished my residency in New York, I went back to Albany to do a two-year fellowship in reconstructive plastic surgery, and then, the next year, I did a one-year fellowship in hand and microvascular surgery at the University of Pittsburgh.

My attraction to the field grew during my fellowship there, but I still didn't know exactly what part of it I would work in, whether I wanted to be an academician or have a private practice. But then Dr. Tom Rees made it easy for me. He was the head of the plastic surgery department at Manhattan Eye, Ear and Throat Hospital, and he was in Pittsburgh when I was presenting a paper at a meeting. He liked my paper and asked me out for a drink, and while we were talking, he convinced me to go back to New York to spend a day at Manhattan Eye and Ear, and if I liked it, to take a fellowship. I already had a job offer from the University of Pittsburgh. One day, as I was trying to decide whether to take it, I was stopped at a red light in my rickety old Saab. This guy pulls up next to me in a gleaming Ferrari. I looked at him and realized that I'd never drive a car like that if I took an academic job.

I spent that day in New York and decided to move back, mainly because of Rees. He was irresistible. Through him I learned more about both this specialty's aesthetic and its human side. Rees operated on kings and movie stars, but he was no snob. He treated the man who pushed the broom around the hospital with the same respect he treated celebrities. He was at the top of the profession, but he was secure with himself. He became my role model. Especially in contrast to the cowboy cardiac and neurosurgeons.

I also learned that plastic surgeons tend to be happy, satisfied people. Intense, but happy. Egotistical, but any good surgeon has to be. You have to be logical and decisive. An internist might say, "Let's see, I think I'll put you on twenty-five milligrams and see how you do. Call me in three days." Surgeons can't do that. You have to act. Now. No hesitation.

Pause on the operating table and you could wind up looking at a corpse.

When I finished with the last fellowship, in 1988, I was thirty-three years old, and my formal education was complete, with the relentless training and sleepless nights behind me. I had to decide what to do, and where. For a while, I thought seriously about going to Beverly Hills. I would share an office with a friend and with my brother. We had introductions to all the right people, and I was promised privileges at Cedar Sinai. But I just didn't feel comfortable in LA. I came back, still unsure of what I wanted to do. I moonlighted in New York for six months, thinking about whether to go the academic route or set up a practice. Although I admit that the Ferrari did have an impact on me, money wasn't the real issue. The thing is, I love to operate, and as an academician I wouldn't have had as much opportunity to do so.

So I went the only way I could go: into practice. I didn't really want to work for someone else, which is probably a good thing, because that's not how plastic surgeons set themselves up in Manhattan. Older doctors don't hire younger doctors. There are few partnerships or groups. That meant I couldn't just go out and get a job in an established practice. I had no money to speak of. With my dwindling savings, I rented office space from an internist on East Eighty-ninth Street, printed up business cards, and started sending out letters to the doctors I'd trained with. If you ever need anyone to cover for you, I told them, I'm here. It didn't hurt that I'd been trained by the surgeons at NYU, either.

Established surgeons left town on weekends and needed younger doctors to take care of their patients if emergencies arose. They also needed to refer the simpler jobs, like sewing up cuts or resetting broken noses. As a result, I slowly began to get referrals. One of the smartest things I did, in retrospect, was treat children—kids who fell and needed stitches to minimize scarring, things like that. I got to know the mothers, and when they saw that I took good care of their children, they remembered me when they wanted cosmetic injections, or a mole removed, or a facelift. It was hardly a glamorous way to start out, but everyone who has succeeded knows you have to start small. At that stage, exposure is everything.

After a year, I had enough money to rent my own office, on East Sixty-fifth Street. For about five years I made a decent living, but I worked my ass off. I saw patients from eight A.M. to eight P.M., Monday through Saturday. On Sunday mornings I often took the bus to the office, where I spent hours typing up thank-you notes to doctors who'd referred patients to me. Steadily, the practice grew. I still worked hard, but I had enough money to replace the hated Saab with a BMW.

And then, in 2000, I found space at 983 Park Avenue, near Eighty-third Street. After renovating, I moved in in February 2001. Park Avenue is the holy grail for plastic surgeons and patients. Before, patients would confess to Lorraine that they liked me, but they wondered why I wasn't on Park Avenue. Wasn't I good enough?

Well, finally I was. Really, there was nothing magic about my arrival there. Patients who liked me and my skills referred their friends, and the practice grew exponentially. Patients come from abroad, from the suburbs, from the city, and in many cases from the neighborhood, with one of America's highest concentrations of the seriously wealthy. I remove a cancerous mole from a CEO's face, and I know he'll be checking me out for his wife's face-lift.

I feel sorry for young plastic surgeons starting out today. Competition is fiercer than ever. Although there are many more people getting plastic surgery, there are also more doctors who can accommodate their needs. Doctors who can't take the competition in New York move to smaller cities, where it may be easier to establish a practice.

I usually can instantly tell who will make it and who won't. Not long ago, as I was walking out of the hospital at seven-twenty A.M. after seeing patients, one of the surgical fellows was strolling in. When I get to the hospital before a resident or a fellow, that's not a good sign. The head of surgery at NYU used to tell us that even if you're not smart, work hard. Any surgeon who doesn't work extra hard in the beginning will never be really successful.

You can't stroll.

You have to run.

My first employee was Lorraine, and she took over all of the business and paperwork, which I hate doing. She's incredibly friendly to all patients, which is crucial. (And incredibly loving to me, which makes her a fantastic wife.) We work together well, and I think that's partly because we don't act married when we're at work. We have totally separate jobs. And when we get home, we might talk a little about how the day went, but then it's over, and we become a couple rather than doctor and office manager.

Lorraine has done a great job of keeping the office well functioning over the years, which is no minor thing. The welcoming atmosphere in an office is as important as a doctor's skills. Prospective patients are likely to check out two or three other doctors and make their final decision based on many factors.

Nor can you succeed only by having the right credentials and a way with a scalpel. Patients are paying hefty fees with their own money, with no hope of reimbursement from their insurance companies, so they can go to any doctor they choose. They want service. And service with a smile. My office staff has to be top-notch, attentive, competent, welcoming, and sparkly, because patients want—and deserve—that kind of atmosphere.

The receptionist is particularly important. If she isn't instantly welcoming, patients will walk away before they even meet me. Building a good office staff is never easy. We have had loyal, hardworking people who become like family. But we've also had our share of disasters.

One secretary was sweet as pie on the surface, but underneath she was as sour as an unripe persimmon. At that time, we had a very wealthy, high-profile patient from France. E-mail didn't yet exist, so this patient would fax us questions, and we would fax back answers. Or at least I thought we were answering. One day Lorraine opened a letter that was addressed to me, marked personal and confidential. (I never open any of the mail; Lorraine shows me what I need to see.) The letter was a shock: "Dear Dr. Lorenc. If I had known you were this type of doctor, I would never have had surgery with you." She went on and on about how inappropriate my office staff's behavior was and then said, please see attached.

Attached was a fax from our secretary, telling the patient she was demanding and difficult. Lorraine read it, got up from her desk, went to the reception area, and fired her. We sent the patient flowers with a long note from me, explaining that it was a mistake and that the person responsible had been fired. To this day I have no idea why that secretary went crazy with this patient. Perhaps the patient had been obnoxious or too direct. It didn't matter. This is a service business, which means that the customer is always right, unless it's a matter of medical judgment and treatment.

Some patient services are less obvious but equally important. Patients don't want to be told that their surgery won't be until three P.M. and that they'll have to spend the day in the hospital, thirsty, hungry, and waiting.

Getting the desirable early morning surgery slots at Manhattan Eye and Ear is one of the office jobs critical to patient contentment. Luckily, we have our connections. Without them, my practice would suffer.

So I've got my staff together. Finally. I like the academic work too. I've written many papers and frequently make presentations at conferences. It's time-consuming and expensive, but it keeps me in contact with other plastic surgeons, and sometimes I learn something new or get new patient referrals. If someone asks about different approaches to a forehead lift, I can say that I helped develop a certain procedure and would be happy to send some of my articles about this subject. It all helps.

I've heard older doctors say that patients now prefer younger doctors. I don't know if that's true. But if it is, it means it's even more important to keep up with current developments. I hate looking stupid. I never want to be in the situation where I'm the old guy who doesn't know a new technique, or be asked a question in the OR that I can't answer. Being on staff at NYU, where I teach residents and fellows, is critical. I lecture to the residents several times a year.

I also watch surgeries performed by my peers. We all do. Or at least the best of us do—even the best of the best want to keep learning. Doctoring is an ongoing process.

Sixteen years into it, my practice is secure, and I can have a life. I can turn down cases I don't want. If I'm out to dinner with friends and a pediatrician calls, I can make a referral to a younger plastic surgeon I like. I don't have to jump up and run out to fix every laceration as I did when I started out. Of course, there are exceptions. I always treat the children of friends, or the children of people who have been patients for a long time. It's been a long, long process to bring me to this point.

The top plastic surgeons who seem so glamorous now all worked like dogs when they started out too. The amount of work you do—as well as the *kind* of work you do—is often incomprehensible to a layperson. The intensity, the hours, the responsibility, and then on top of that creating a business, taking care of your employees, and maybe having a date once in a blue moon. It was tough. But brutal training's got to be done to weed out those who can take it from those who can't.

And I am not complaining!

Which is why when I'm asked why I charge so much, I can reply that I'm not getting paid solely for the three hours it takes to do surgery. You're paying me for the years I spent in school, the years I spent as an intern and a resident, the years I continued my training, and the fact that I will always continue to train. You're paying for the monumental effort I made so you can trust me implicitly in the operating room.

When you get to the top and you have a lucrative boutique practice, you've earned it. You know that you're good, and you know that all the hard work is finally paying off. And if you don't believe you are the best, doing the best job possible, you shouldn't be doing it.

For those of us who love what we do, the most fundamental aspect of our success is making people happy. Once, an elderly Sicilian man named Giovanni, who had immigrated to the United States, came to me with a lesion on his head. As a Medicare patient, Giovanni hadn't exactly received stellar care—he'd had this lesion for several years, and his doctor told him to put steroid cream on it. The steroids were useless, because the biopsy I immediately ordered revealed squamous cell carcinoma, the kind that could go straight to his brain. I told him we needed to find a neurosurgeon and have immediate surgery. It was a huge procedure. The neurosurgeon removed part of his skull, then I did the reconstruction of his face. After radiation and chemotherapy, he did well.

Afterward, Giovanni and his wife sent us pastries and holiday cards every year. About two years later, early one morning, Giovanni and his wife were waiting for me outside my office. Perplexed, I asked what I could do for him, and he said he had something for me. In tears, he handed me an envelope. Even more perplexed, I opened it. There was five thousand dollars in cash inside. "Take it, please, Doctor," Giovanni said. "The Medicare people never paid you enough for saving my life."

My eyes filled with tears too. I told them of course that I couldn't take it, but that I understood what it meant to him. That I, too, was an immigrant, and I knew it had to have taken him years to save that kind of money, and that I had been fully reimbursed by the pleasure I took in seeing him get better.

Most cases are not that dramatic, but there are many other grateful patients who make my days worthwhile. Patients feel and look better, they get compliments, and often their true selves begin to emerge.

A successful stockbroker had suffered with polio as a child, and it atrophied one of his calves. When he came to me, he said that he never thought he would be considering plastic surgery, it seemed so shallow to worry about such things, but his leg made him unbearably self-conscious. He never wanted anyone to see it. I did a calf augmentation for him, and after his last postsurgical visit, he said to me that at age forty-eight, he was wearing shorts for the first time in his life.

A similar change occurred in a woman who was very plain and married to a much older man. She came in originally with a friend who was having her nose done. While she was here, her friend convinced her to talk to me, and she ended up deciding to have a chin implant. We didn't see her for a few months. All of a sudden one day the door opened and this beautiful woman walked in. Lorraine didn't recognize her, but she did remember the voice. The chin implant had given her so much confidence that she went out and had her hair cut short, she started wearing makeup, and she bought beautiful clothes. She looked completely different, although frankly she had had a very small surgical procedure. The change in her was not surgical. It was primarily psychological, and it led to these immense physical changes.

I find it very gratifying to give patients what they want. I don't tell people they need to change, but if they say they're unhappy, and they want guidance, I give it to them. They may not "need" surgery from a life-threatening point of view, but it's *their* point of view that matters. If I think I can help them, and the procedure they want is aesthetically reasonable as well as medically safe, there's no reason not to do it.

Plastic surgery should be life-enhancing.

And I'm all for enhancing life.

Five

MUSIC TO MY EARS, OR I LOVE SURGERY

"I'M MARY."

"Excuse me?" I asked.

"Mary," the patient replied. "Haven't you heard of me? Mary. As in Peter, Paul, and Mary. Look—that's me here. *Mary.* Next to Peter."

I'd met "Mary" during my mandatory psych rotation in medical school. Every morning she'd bring me the album cover and show me the picture. And then she'd start to sing.

She certainly didn't sound very much like the real Mary. But she did help me realize that psychiatry was not going to be my specialty, even though I would learn soon enough that a healthy dollop of psychiatric understanding is an integral part of any plastic surgeon's practice, particularly when dealing with either deluded or narcissistic patients. (Don't worry, I'll get to them later.) I don't have the patient, constantly empathetic personality necessary to best help psychiatric patients, I knew. Most surgeons don't. That's why we operate. I was always interested in doing something that was either it's this way or it's not. Black or white. Open and shut. You go in and do it, and it's done.

Sometimes when my wife is trying to deal with a million things clamoring for her attention, she tells me that I'm lucky because I get to go in the operating room and have no stress.

She's right. I love doing surgery, I love thinking about surgery.

I love doing surgery so much that when I'm operating, I'm pumped up with adrenaline and utterly focused on my patient. Every time I pick up a scalpel, I get a rush. Every patient is different, and I won't know what I'm going to find until I get in there. That makes every day a new challenge. Procedures I've done a thousand times never become routine.

Think about it. Why would anybody let you take her face apart? It's the ultimate trust. I even see it as more powerful than someone who puts herself into the hands of a cardiac surgeon. In most cases, cardiac surgery is not optional. Aesthetic surgery always is. My patients are giving me liberty to rip their faces off and put them all back together again.

As long as I don't make them look like Humpty Dumpty. Or Joan Rivers.

I never drink the night before surgery. It has nothing to do with my concern about my physical dexterity, or having a stable hand. Drinking cuts down on mental acuity. Reflexes are slower. That doesn't mean I don't go out for drinks with my friends on evenings that don't precede surgery. Of course I do. I don't tend to have emergencies, so I don't have to worry about being called in for a critical operation.

The need for plastic surgery began after World War One, when horribly wounded war veterans crowded the wards in veterans' hospitals. Surgeons helped fix some of these difficult wounds, and worked on reconstruction techniques for some of the most devastating scars. Reconstruction work is as much a part of a plastic surgeon's repertoire as knowing how to slice off a dowager's jowls. I also studied microvascular surgery, which involves massive reconstruction. For example, to remove a tumor in the esophagus, you'd take a piece of the small intestine, put it in the neck, then reconnect everything. That's complicated beyond belief, and I don't do that kind of work now, because it involves a team of surgeons, working in a hospital, with constant follow-up and a large support staff. I prefer to fly solo.

But whatever the procedure, many people entertain the misperception that plastic surgery is bullshit surgery. The procedures are swift and painless, and results immediate.

No surgery that can wind up killing a patient is bullshit surgery! Even though I meet with patients for the initial consultation, and then again before surgery, explaining in gory detail what to expect so they aren't shocked by the pain and the bruises and the swelling, many of them refuse to listen or take me seriously. Until after the procedure, when they can't believe how swollen they are and how crummy they feel.

Sometimes my honesty doesn't work out so well. Once I told Mr. Macho Investment Banker what would happen during his face-lift, and he passed out. He made such a loud noise that the nurse came screaming.

Another patient had breast implants ten years before. They'd been put above the muscle, which is not the ideal placement. She needed surgery to have them taken out and put under the muscle, and she also needed a breast-lift. She told me she was taking an antidepressant, and I told her she must stop taking it two weeks before the surgery.

She came in, she was prepped, and she was given anesthesia. Everything was fine. But the second I made the incision she started bleeding all over the place. I stopped the bleeding and made a new incision. She bled more copiously, dripping down my pants, onto my shoes, pooling on the floor. I silently swore and kept going. I was already committed; I had made the incision. If I thought her life was in danger I would have packed the wound and stopped, but she wasn't in mortal danger. The surgery took twice as long as usual. I was furious because her bleeding was due to the fact that she hadn't stopped taking her antidepressant as instructed.

Immediately after the surgery, she was fine. A few months later she came in, and when I saw her I knew right away she'd had a mild stroke. I told her that if she didn't stop taking the antidepressant she would die, because one of its possible side effects is stroke, but she wouldn't listen. I called her husband and told him his wife was risking her life and helped him find her a new internist and psychiatrist. She needed help.

I do about half my surgeries at Manhattan Eye and Ear on East Sixty-fourth Street, where most of the top plastic surgeons work, and the other half in my office. The operating room in my office is certified under the American Association for Accreditation of Ambulatory Surgery Facilities as a surgical center, so it is ready for any emergency. Office ORs are easier for doctors and less expensive for patients, as the room fee is cheaper, usually half the cost of what a hospital charges. The office operating room is a bit more relaxed, and patients get more attention. They are the total focus of the staff, and they go home with a private duty nurse. That's not the case in the hospital, where one nurse has to deal with many patients.

Surgery usually starts early, around eight A.M., because patients have had to stop eating and drinking at midnight, and I don't like to keep them waiting any longer than necessary. By the time I see the patient, he or she has already changed into a robe. As soon as I finish my initial work, the anesthesiologist begins. A crucial part of the surgery happens in these ten or fifteen minutes, because I draw the surgery I am about to do. Using an erasable pen, I make every mark on the skin that the scalpel will follow.

Anesthesia is as critical to the surgical process as my skill with the scalpel, because going under sedation is where real damage can occur. How quickly do patients go under? How smoothly do they wake up? That makes all the difference. One reason I like doing surgery in my office is that I work with the same anesthesiologists, either Tim or Steve, and we've become a comfortable team. And they're fun. My surgical nurse, Lolita, hands me everything I need during surgery, and after sixteen years together, she can practically read my mind. She is a dream to have by my side in the operating room.

This kind of teamwork helps me, as I do only the kinds of surgeries where I know I can deliver the very best result possible. I'm not interested in doing a surgery if it's only an occasional procedure. If I'm not going to be the best, I refer the patient to someone else.

Surgery is never boring. I'm always thinking about how I can perfect what I do, how smoothly and quickly I can perform every step, even something as mundane as sewing the stitches. I concentrate on the motions and on the fluidity. I try to be better each time I operate. And I think that way even when I'm approaching nonsurgical procedures. Each time I inject Restylane or Botox, I try to make it smoother and better. You have to present these challenges to yourself in your work.

Otherwise you become a slug.

Some surgeries take more concentration than others. In one difficult case, a woman involved at a high level in politics was having eyelid surgery. Her lower lid drooped slightly from a prior procedure she'd had done five years earlier, when too much fat had been taken out. I had to be very careful not to add to the droopiness. I took fat and skin out of her upper eyelid and then worked on the ligament to try to reduce the droopiness in the lower lid. My focus was so intense I completely lost track of everything else. I knew how important this woman was, how knowledgeable. And, let's be frank, I also knew she could refer me a lot of new patients. If I botched the job, she could just as easily tell her friends that Lorenc is a schmuck.

When I operate in the hospital rather than in my office, I may work with different anesthesiologists and nurses each time, and visiting fellows and other doctors often stop in. Sometimes they scrub in and work with me. There's only one constant in my surgeries in the hospital: I always have music playing.

Much to their surprise and sometimes to the dismay of my colleagues, I love blasting songs by the Allman Brothers. Gregg and I became good friends after he was referred to me by Dickie Betts, his musical partner at the time, and I did a procedure on him. Backstage after a concert years ago, Gregg put his arm around me and announced, "This is my plastic surgeon." It was on Page 6 of the *New York Post* the next day.

Of course that's not the reason I like him. He's a truly nice man, smart and savvy. You'd never think he was a former drug-addicted rock and roller whose tempestuous marriage to Cher was tabloid fodder for years. He's thrilled with what I did for him, and he looks great. Not *done*. Just relaxed. And I still get a kick out of remembering how I used to play Allman Brothers songs on the pizza-joint jukebox when I was in high school.

Anyway, the Allman Brothers are a great band to do suction to. Gregg told me he's got a cardiac surgeon pal who cracks open every chest to the strains of "Jessica." He's got good taste. That's the song I like to play when I'm doing liposuction. There's something about the beat—it's perfect for the rhythm of pushing the cannula in and out, in and out.

In addition to music, there's plenty of chitchat with my colleagues while we're working in the OR. I find it relaxing to talk during surgery but not when I'm working on the muscles during a face-lift. Then, even I shut up. I'm concentrating deeply, working right next to the nerves. The room becomes absolutely quiet. Once I finish that section, though, it's back to rock and roll.

The truth is, the operating room is our office. When we have to work hard, we do, but we also banter and joke and gossip and talk about current events, accompanied by the steady *beep beep beep* of the equipment monitoring the patient's vital signs. Once the patient is really out, we can talk about anything and not be heard.

"Did I tell you the story of how I almost got bounced from Bellevue?" I said one day as I began working on the left cheek of a woman getting a face-lift. "I was a second-year resident, the surgical consult in the ER. That day there was a disaster, a four-alarm fire. I went out with the crew in the mobile emergency rescue vehicle. We called it the MERV. It's as big as a bus, but there's an operating room inside. You can crack a chest in there. So we rode down to SoHo, then stood around having coffee and doughnuts from the Salvation Army. It was two hours of wasted time. On the way back, driving on the FDR, the EMS technician says to me, 'Hey, Doc, you wanna drive?'

"Well, how could I turn that down? So I sit down, and I'm driving, and I put the siren on and the lights. It was great. So I get back to the ER and tell all my friends, 'Hey, I drove the bus, it was really cool.' Two days later I got paged by Frank Spencer's office, he was the chief of surgery. You got called in there only when there was trouble. His secretary was named Honey—something you never forget. I went in thinking, what the hell did I do? And then Honey asked me if I drove the EMS bus on the FDR a couple of nights ago.

" 'Yes, I did. On the way back from a fire.'

"Honey waved a piece of paper at me. 'Here's a letter from the nurse who was in the bus with you, and she claims you put everyone's life in danger.' Then she winked. 'Frank's not going to see this, but you have to behave yourself in the future. Understand?'

"I nodded, deeply shaken, and eternally grateful to Honey. That nurse could have ruined my career with one letter. So when I left Honey's office, the first thing I did was line up all the surgical residents, all of my buddies, and tell them what she'd done. Whenever that nurse walked by, they would make crude comments. Am I proud of that now? No. But at the time I was a selfish brat and I was furious that she tried to do me in behind my back."

Tim laughed, and Lolita rolled her eyes.

I looked down at my handiwork near my patient's hairline. "I'm sure you've seen women where the hairline is up to here," I went on, gesturing to her skull. "You know who was a perfect example? Martha Graham."

"She had a tuft on the top of her head," Tim said.

A knack with hair and hairlines is one of the key things I try to teach the residents. Although sometimes I'm not sure it can be taught. It's more of an instinct. When I see a resident at work, within minutes I can tell if he or she will be good.

The woman I was working on had lovely skin, and I thought she'd get a very good result when I finished with her. As I pulled the skin away from her face, bloody gauze hung out of a hole by her ear. I had completely snipped the skin away from its base, called undermining. I did liposuction under her chin and tightened the muscles of her face. Before I started to put her back together, I carefully checked her, cauterizing to ensure there'd be no bleeding when the skin was closed. I pulled the skin up by the ear and cut around the ear, throwing the leftover skin toward Lolita.

Surgery is not pretty.

Then I sewed that side back up, a process that sounds simple but is anything but.

When I get to the sewing, it looks like I'm doing it without thinking, but of course I'm not. It took years to figure out exactly the right amount of tension for the closure. I have to make the skin blanch just a little bit, because it loosens after the surgery, and if I don't do that, it will be too loose. But if I make it too tight the scar will be noticeable. You can't start out going too far. You have to work up to it. It's a judgment call, honed by years of experience. Basically, you have to screw up to learn it, first by watching, then by assisting, then by doing it yourself. I do a better face-lift today than fifteen years ago. Not that they were bad, but these are better.

By ten-thirty, the right side of her face was done. I put in the drains, sliding a tube through one hole and out the other. Tim gave her some more sedative because she was starting to move around a little on the table, which could be disastrous. We don't want her to feel anything. And we really don't want her to move when I'm using a scalpel.

Although I constantly look at the patient as I work on first one side of her face and then the other, my prior planning is the most crucial part. During surgery, the face becomes swollen, and if I go into it depending solely on visual signs I can make a mistake.

I've had writers and medical students who want to watch surgery. Sometimes they pass out or have to leave the room. It can take a while to get accustomed to surgery. But once you are, believe me, it's nothing. For us, peeling skin off faces and opening up bodies is the most normal thing in the world. A patient getting a breast reduction looks like an open pack of hamburger on the table. Once her skin is rolled down and there's nothing but innards sitting on a chest, you'd think there's no way to put her back together again. Somehow, it all manages to come together.

I get Botox, but I've never had surgery. Only because I don't have the desire for it. Yet.

But if I need it ten years from now, I'll take care of it in a second. Most plastic surgeons have worked on their wives, and I'm no exception. It's made her even more empathetic to our patients' anxieties and post-op healing. And the procedures merely enhanced her natural beauty.

Doing surgery on my mother was something else.

Thirteen years ago my mother wanted to have her face and eyes done. I told her to go to Dr. Baker or Dr. Aston, but she wouldn't have it. "Who's going to do a better job on me than you?" she asked. I couldn't argue with that logic, so I finally agreed to do it.

My mother was prepped, and I'd marked up her face. The chief anesthesiologist, Peter, put her out into twilight sleep; generally we don't use a general anesthesia. I was sitting at the head of the table. After the patient is sedated, I infiltrate the face with a numbing medicine.

"Peter, can I start?" I asked, and he said yes. I looked at my hand, holding an enormous syringe, and it was shaking. I looked at Peter and the nurses, and I told myself, This is pretty fucking crazy. There is no way I can operate on my mother. But I didn't want to look like a fool—I *hate* looking like a fool—so I tried to control the shaking. I couldn't.

I took a deep breath and somehow managed to put the needle right under the skin. More important, I quickly realized my mother was not reacting to pain. My hand became rock steady. From that point on, she was just another patient. The surgery was perfect.

I told my mother about my shaking hand later, and she cried. My mom, one tough cookie, was in tears. She knew my apprehension had been a primordial protective mechanism. I hadn't wanted to hurt the woman who gave me life.

Thank goodness my mother was ecstatic after surgery. But I wouldn't recommend operating on your mother. It's an unnecessary stress.

And let's face it. Life is already stressful enough without slicing open your mother.

Six

THE PARK AVENUE POSSE: COMPETING ANY WAY POSSIBLE

ALL PLASTIC SURGEONS ARE EGOTISTICAL.

We have to train incredibly hard. We have to work incredibly hard. We must be driven. Of course we're egotistical.

But our egos are a matter of degree. Some of my colleagues start to believe in their skills to such an extent that it becomes nothing more than pure unadulterated bullshit. They think they can operate in a parallel universe, one free from censure and filled with their own grandiosity. They start to believe their own publicity.

Until they mess up.

Even among the surgical cowboys, plastic surgery has become breathtakingly competitive. For one thing, getting reimbursed and doing all the mind-numbing paperwork for the insurance companies is a nightmare for most doctors. Unlike them, however, aesthetic surgeons aren't dependent on the ever-lower fees allowed by insurance companies, because we don't generally do procedures, except for reconstruction after cancer, for instance, that involve insurance. Our patients come to us because they want what we have to offer, and they're willing to pay for it.

And they're going to shop around for it too.

Not having to deal with insurance—and being paid large sums of cash for elective procedures—is a very attractive proposition for doctors. And thanks to the simple fact that any doctor licensed to do surgery can do surgery, guess who's doing plastic surgery? Eye doctors, dermatologists, gynecologists, podiatrists. You name it, they're doing it. It's perfectly legal.

It's also perfectly insane. No one requires that these doctors be well trained to do the procedures. Some of these doctors start doing complicated liposuction and eye jobs after just a weekend course. That is not exactly the same level of expertise as someone who's board certified in plastic surgery and has spent years training for that certification.

But hey, if you want your gynecologist to suck out your flab after she gives you a Pap smear, be my guest.

Just remember: I'm not about to deliver your baby.

And for another thing, because we're now competing with non–plastic surgeons, the pressure is intense to present ourselves as having the newest, the best, the most unusual, the laser du jour that will make patients sit up and take notice.

Actually, as I've said already, what gets written up as "new and fabulous" usually isn't. What doctors claim to have "discovered" isn't any new "discovery." The surgical wheel is not reinvented every day. PR does play a huge part in the hype.

What becomes a problem, though, is that a lot of this PR, by both surgeons and the media, precedes any real science. People currently talk about lasers as the second coming. It's nonsense. Lasers are pulses of intense light that tighten the skin. They are perfect for smoothing out scarred or lightly wrinkled skin, but they can't replace a scalpel. They can't lift sagging skin that is making the chin disappear. What they can do is occasionally burn skin, leaving irreparable damage in the form of hideous scarring.

Furthermore, it's usually not helpful to a practice when a young-buck doctor claims to have found the newest and best way to do something. I understand the temptation to brag or sell yourself, because a doctor fresh out of residency and drowning in debt is tempted to do anything to get patients. But the top plastic surgeons are something of a clique, to put it bluntly, and they find ways to punish doctors who go too far while whoring for patients.

Not long ago, there was a resident who finished the NYU program and was so arrogant he thought he was a professor before he was even out. Right away, he came up with this gimmick to jump-start his practice. He was doing Botox "to go," taking Botox in a refrigerator—you have to keep it cold—and an assistant and going to hotels, bars, and gyms to inject people. He was just two weeks out of his residency, and he must have hired a PR person to get the word out. Botox to go is not considered proper behavior. The American Society of Plastic Surgeons makes it clear in its pronouncements that Botox should only be administered in an appropriately equipped and staffed medical office. I predict he won't be getting board certified in the near future. He will eventually, but starting with a stunt like that was a really bad idea.

We compete with the new, and we compete with each other, in all kinds of ways, some subtle and some obvious. Thanks to our aforementioned naturally ego-driven, inherently godlike personalities. We all know we're the best.

But who is the best of the best?

Let's say one of my esteemed colleagues gives me some advice. I have no way of knowing his motives. Is he trying to help me, or hurt me? When I started out, many doctors told me that it made no sense to sew up little kids' busted faces, and they urged me not to waste my time doing that. But I knew in my gut it would translate into more business, and I was right. I often see the parents of children I took care of years before. Were those "helpful" doctors trying to steer me wrong? Who knows.

Some doctors also, subtly or not so subtly, bad-mouth other doctors. I don't press for names of other surgeons my patients have seen for consultations. Really, I don't want to know, because I don't want to have to say anything about my colleagues. Patients love to gossip. Word gets around.

It's a very small world, and the Park Avenue Posse is an even smaller part of it.

There are only four thousand board-certified plastic surgeons in the United States. Of those, probably twelve hundred participate in professional meetings. And of those, probably only two or three hundred give presentations and regularly take part in research and writing. In the entire country there are probably about a hundred excellent plastic surgeons. But on the whole, many more than that have good training and can do a good job.

But they're not part of our elite posse.

So, getting back to bad-mouthing, one patient told me she'd gone to three surgeons for consultations, and when she asked one about me, the doctor said, "You shouldn't go to him. He doesn't know as much about breast surgery as I do."

That's a ridiculous way to compete.

If I were a patient and a doctor started trashing another doctor, I'd walk right out. I'd never trust any doctor who has to prove himself or herself with every patient by belittling others. I don't let myself get drawn into this sort of thing—because you never know if a patient might be making the whole thing up.

So when patients ask, "Why should I come to you? Why shouldn't I go to Dr. X or Dr. Y?" I have a standard answer. If the surgeon is a complete shyster, or I perceive him to be a shyster, I say, "I have never heard of him."

Even though, of course, I have. Patients pick up on what that means.

If I consider the doctor to be a reputable surgeon, I say, "Dr. Y is a good surgeon. I know him personally, and I don't think you can make a mistake by going with either of us."

Park Avenue plastic surgeons don't usually socialize with one another, at least not in New York. If I go to a party and there's another plastic surgeon there, our guard goes up. We smile through our teeth even as we look warily at one another. We're not consciously out trawling for patients, but you never know. So how could we be friends, really?

Surgeons do socialize at the conventions, but it's all very general. You know, how-is-everything-great-how's-it-going-with-you. You don't go into detail. Occasionally we talk about technique, but really it's more like nondescript chitchat when surgeons get together. We're far too competitive and protective of our turf to risk letting any juicy tidbits slide out. Not surprisingly, the surgeons I consider snakes, especially those who consistently belittle or derogate others, are a must to avoid. It can be tricky. Our competitive nature is so strong that some of us joke that we'd have to go out of town if we wanted face-lifts. Would I trust someone who'd love to get his hands on my practice? I don't think so.

Slices surgeons take from one another are far more subtle than those that would be wielded with a scalpel. When I was just starting to be truly successful, one of the top plastic surgeons told me I wasn't charging enough for surgery. So I told Lorraine to raise the prices. Almost immediately, business started slowing down. With the new rates, I was charging almost as much as the top guys, and I realized that if patients decided to pay that much, they might as well pay a bit more and get someone better known.

Lorraine was convinced they told me to raise my prices to undermine the practice. I'll never know. Prices are difficult to assess. You have to continually raise them as you get more successful so that you don't become overwhelmed with patients, but of course you have to be careful not to raise them too high. People do price-shop and see multiple doctors, and they come in quoting the other estimates. This keeps us abreast of what our competition charges.

Naturally, we compete on prices, something that can have both good and bad consequences for patients. Lower prices are often available, and even well-established doctors sometimes have flexible fees. To a certain extent, a fee is what the market will bear, and the market varies from person to person in some offices, although not in mine. I've heard of doctors who set their fee schedule according to how a patient looks. If she looks really rich, she's charged more. There is nothing to regulate that.

My advice is to dress down and keep your jewelry in the safe when you go to see a Park Avenue surgeon.

When patients don't show up for their scheduled surgery, it's not because they're nervous. It's because they got a better price somewhere else. Sometimes they don't even bother to call. Once Lorraine called to schedule a patient with the hospital, and the booking clerk told her the patient was already set up to be operated on by another doctor. It happens to all of us. A famous singer was scheduled to be operated on by an equally famous plastic surgeon, who found out he'd been ditched for the competition only when he was in the hospital and saw her on another surgeon's operating table.

Another thing to think about is the enormous changes in plastic surgery over the years. Top doctors must keep constantly learning to stay abreast of new techniques. At professional conferences, papers are presented and new ideas are discussed; some of them are actual courses. Sometimes my surgeries are videotaped and shown at the meetings so younger doctors can learn the techniques. That's always a kick.

In the beginning, I used to learn a lot at meetings, but the material quickly became repetitive. Too many doctors taking credit for things they didn't actually invent, as well as a lot of inflated claims for "new" techniques. Many presentations are no more than individuals who want to hear themselves talk. I think they ultimately do a huge disservice; they cheat young plastic surgeons who pay their money and want to learn. Recently, a group of Brazilian surgeons did a presentation about mini–tummy tucks. Their patients were twenty years old. That's right, *twenty*. The results were fantastic, but of course these ladies didn't need any surgery to begin with. To me, that's insane. I resent it.

I didn't always feel this way. When I first went into practice, I was excited about meeting everyone and seeing everything. But it's easy to get disillusioned after years of seeing the same stuff over and over, especially when much of it isn't truthful. Okay, perhaps not truthful is too harsh. What looks good and what doesn't look good is entirely subjective, and standards of beauty are impossible to quantify. At one meeting, a doctor was talking about the need to inject fat around the eye to restore a youthful look. He showed before and after pictures, and I shook my head. I didn't see any difference, yet he was standing there trying to convince everybody that this technique was wonderful. Another surgeon talked about how he was putting big cheek implants into patients and doing face-lifts that way. He showed photos. His patients looked different, all right. But to me, they didn't look better.

What gets my goat is that we all get lumped together at conferences— the best doctors and the self-serving opportunists with about as much finesse as a charging rhino.

There are turf issues too. Sometimes they spill over into public places, usually after one doctor takes too much credit for something and pisses someone off. A few years ago, Dr. Alan Matarasso, a prominent Park Avenue surgeon, gave a report in a meeting in Los Angeles about his use of a technique he called the short scar face-lift. In his presentation he neglected to give credit to Dr. Daniel Baker, a senior and at least as prominent surgeon who had performed that procedure countless times himself. Dr. Baker was furious when he heard about it. Their feud was covered by the media, Baker trying to protect his turf and accusing Matarasso of trying to take it. In truth, no single surgeon developed the technique—I can think of several others who had been using it—and it is silly to say that one did.

Here's a perfect example of how subtle our competition can get: A man named Chris came to see me, age forty-nine, relatively good-looking, fit and trim, dressed casually with smart, good taste. He sat down with a memo pad, and I thought, oh no, this is going to be torture, as he started talking about his eyelids and his brow. He went into minute detail about technique, asking me things such as, "How do you approach the mid face? How do you suspend the malar fat pad?" Those are not questions most patients usually ask.

Then he asked if I do the deep plane face-lift, and I said I did it on occasion, where it was appropriate. I explained that I was involved in a study in 1992 that proved that there was no difference between a standard SMAS face-lift and the deep plane one but that there were more significant risks to the deep plane lift. It involves going underneath the muscle, so the chance of injury to the nerve is higher. Patients, however, thought doing something "deep" was going to be better. Not according to science. Preference for the deep plane lift was based on a PR campaign by the doctors who did it.

Chris nodded, then asked about nerve injuries and what technique I would use on his eyelids.

After I explained, I asked, "What do you do for a living? Obviously, you've done your homework."

He said he'd recently sold a multibillion-dollar business, and he was now enjoying life. He wanted work done on his face, and he wanted the best. He'd already interviewed many doctors.

"I've interviewed nine plastic surgeons. You're the tenth. I saw Aston and Baker before I came to you."

I was amazed. I had never seen someone do that much research.

"Dr. Baker told me that the endoscopic brow-lift doesn't work," he went on. "How do you respond to that?"

Touché. He knew that I had been one of the pioneers in that technique, and that I use it all the time.

"Your question to Dr. Baker," I replied, "needs to be how often does he perform an endoscopic brow-lift."

When our meeting was over, Chris said he wanted copies of some of my articles, which I sent to him.

Finally, he asked the question so many people ask. "Why should I come to you?"

"I don't think you can go wrong with any of the surgeons you've mentioned," I said carefully, giving him my standard answer. "They're all in a separate class from everyone else. It's strictly a personal decision."

He thanked me and left. The very strangest thing was, I never saw him again, and I never heard whether he booked surgery with anyone else at Manhattan Eye and Ear.

And so it goes.

Intensity and competitiveness spill over into other parts of my life. I can't help it. Take one of my best friends, Dickie Betts, the guitar player who used to be in the Allman Brothers band. We were down in Florida on vacation. It was tarpon season, so we got up early in the morning to go fishing, picked up our guide, and got into our boat. We had to go through a series of bridges that had to be opened for us. Dickie gave the signal for the guy to open up the bridges, but the bridge guy was obviously sleeping. Finally, the guy woke up, moving in slow motion. It made Dickie crazy. "I'm gonna bite your fucking head off! You motherfucker! You made me wait!" Dickie screamed at the poor guy.

Mind you, we'd been kept waiting maybe five minutes, but it was five too many for Dickie.

And as soon as we got through all the bridges, Dickie leaned back and smiled. "I'm just a people person," he said.

Like a lot of surgeons I know.

I'm sure each thinks of himself or herself as a "people person" too.

But I can have my moments. When Lorraine and I took our five-year-old son, Paul Jr., to interview for kindergarten, we soon realized it was like getting into an Ivy League school. The tours, the tests, the interviews, the aggravation, the sleepless nights worrying if your child is good enough.

And the kids are five.

When we were interviewing at the Dalton School, one of the best in Manhattan, the woman asked us what we liked to do with our son.

"Rock climbing in Central Park," I said immediately.

"We also like to raise ladybugs in the house with the kids. Central Park is like our backyard," Lorraine added. "We go bird-watching there too."

I held my tongue. We've never gone bird-watching in our lives.

When we were getting ready to leave, the woman said, "You've told me two very impressive things. No one ever told me they go bird-watching. Or that they raise bugs."

Our son got in, but we decided to send him elsewhere.

I love New York.

Seven

JUST SAY NO

NO.

One small leap for me, one giant step for plastic surgeons everywhere. Sometimes, you've just got to say no.

No to those who are unrealistic or irresponsible.

No to those who are impossible to please.

No to those who've already had too many procedures.

No to self-confessed surgery junkies.

No to procedures that I think might be dangerous.

No to products I have doubts about.

No is one of the most important weapons in my arsenal. There is so much hype in the plastic surgery world that patients need a reality check.

They need someone who will say, "No, there is no such thing as a lunch-hour face-lift, and anyone who tells you that is nuts."

"No, having a sixth nose job is not a good idea, because the tiny snip of cartilage you still have left will collapse."

"No. You can't have another face-lift. There are no wrinkles on your face."

"No, I'm sorry, Mr. Jackson, but you do not need to make your nose any smaller."

The only problem with *no*?

There's always going to be another surgeon who'll say *yes*.

No matter how much pressure a patient exerts, no matter how much wheedling and begging, it's important to refuse to give in to what he or she wants if you think it's the wrong decision. Jocelyn Wildenstein, whose plastic surgery was much commented on a few years ago during her divorce, ended up resembling one of the big cats (lion, cheetah, jaguar, you name it) she adored. Her doctor will forevermore be associated with her now famously feline face.

Let me make one particularly important point about *no*. I don't judge my patients, even those who are clearly deluded and in dire need of psychological help. Any plastic surgeon who judges his patients is in the wrong business. For most people who want surgery, there's a good chance that the changes will please them. These are valid decisions. I don't say no to valid decisions.

And as long as patients are in touch with reality, and understand what I can and can't do, I'm willing to help, even if they are a tad neurotic. When I go home at night, I want to be able to sleep like a baby. I don't want any guilt over making bad decisions solely based on greed or competition.

But there is an obvious difference between not judging a healthy, normal patient who wants to look younger or better, and a patient who's crossed the line into an unhealthy *obsession* with looking younger or better.

WHEN SURGERY IS THE LAST THING YOUR PATIENT NEEDS

- She has totally unreasonable expectations. Like, for instance, the woman in her sixties who kept showing me the photo from a magazine of an eighteen-year-old with a beautiful nose.
- He reveals himself to be either obsessive-compulsive or in the grips of body dysmorphic disorder, in which a perceived flaw, such as a tiny scar on his face, is magnified completely out of

proportion to reality. He looks normal but endlessly insists that some aspect of his body is unacceptable. If I take a magnifying glass and I can't see anything, I know that surgery is not the solution. If I don't see it, it's not there. It's only in his head.

- She wants a specific result but isn't willing to go through the process necessary to get there. For instance, if a woman has deep lines between her mouth and nose and doesn't want a face-lift— insisting that she knows best, that Botox will do the trick—she's not being realistic. Realism is a crucial part of the process. No matter what I do, she'll be unhappy.
- He appears to be deaf. He wants something that I can't do, and I tell him that. But he keeps insisting that he wants it. And wants it. And wants it.
- She is convinced that a procedure will instantly change her life.

Often, people see a little line forming, or the beginning of a sag, and they panic. I try to explain that they always have to consider the benefit-to-risk ratio. If it's a big improvement, then it's usually reasonable. If you're overly eager to take on the risk of anesthesia and scarring for only a minor improvement, then it doesn't make sense.

Those are the patients I must say no to. And those are the patients who just don't want to hear it. If a patient says she wants her thighs to be thin and smooth, and she pulls her skin up to make it smooth, I tell her I can't do that . . . but I can give her a better contour. She won't have perfect skin. If she understands that, fine. If she doesn't, I won't do it, and she'll go elsewhere.

When patients want something, they'll push until they get it, even if it means going from doctor to doctor. The saddest cases are the ones where I tell patients to go slowly, that it's important to be conservative, but they don't want to hear it. Some patients absolutely refuse to listen when I tell them what medicine can and cannot do for them. Two women came to see me, both very attractive. They'd had beautifully done face-lifts, and now they wanted liposuction on their thighs. As they were in their late fifties, I had to tell them both that their skins' elasticity simply wasn't good enough, that liposuction would *add* to the dimpling on their thighs, and they would be unhappy with the results.

They weren't pleased with the truth, but I wasn't about to lie. Unfortunately, of course, it would be easy enough to find a surgeon who would. But liposuction can't remove cellulite. Indeed, it can make it worse.

Take Anna. I knew immediately that Anna was trouble. She was only twenty-three, pretty, and to the naked eye just about flawless. But she came in with an almost grim demeanor, wanting to do something about the creases between her mouth and her nose. These lines, the nasolabial folds, are created when the fat pads on the cheeks descend, and they become deeper as people age. Everyone has those creases, except very young children, and nothing can prevent them.

Anna's lines weren't deep, but they bothered her. This was our second meeting; she'd been more than an hour late for her first appointment, and I could talk with her only briefly then. After just a minute, I'd known she was one of those patients I could never please, which makes treating them an exercise in frustration. I know this not by their look, but by the way they ask questions. By their *tone*.

When I was just starting out, I would take on almost every patient who came my way. I didn't know then what I know now: I can't make everyone happy.

I start assessing a new patient the minute she starts talking. I'm asking myself: Does she seem like a stable individual? Will she be able to handle the surgery and the post-op? Are her expectations realistic? Is she asking appropriate questions?

If my radar goes up, and I can tell that a patient's going to be unreasonable, I try never actually to say I'd rather not see him or her. I just have the front desk play very, very hard to get, and say there are no openings for six months. Usually, a patient can get an appointment much more quickly than that.

Getting back to Anna. Normally, she would never have gotten another appointment. But a new receptionist had started working that week, and she had no idea that Anna was difficult. And now here she was, and I walked into the room with a smile on my face. No one wants to see a doctor who looks grim. I always put on a positive face for the patient, no matter what's already gone on that day.

Anna started right in, complaining about her nonexistent lines. I explained how Restylane worked, that it was the best thing on the market for the lines around the mouth, and that in no circumstances should she ever let anyone give her Botox for those lines, because it would give the mouth an artificial, paralyzed look. The idea was simply to fill in the creases, the way grout is used to fill the spaces between tiles.

"Does Restylane ever cause infections?" she asked, which was a legitimate question.

"In the nearly two years I've been using it, I've never seen an infection," I replied.

"But are you *sure* I won't get an infection?" she pressed.

"I can't give you a guarantee. It can still happen no matter what I do."

"What about lumps?"

"Occasionally there might be, but they could be eliminated by massage."

Anna frowned. "Would there be any raised areas? Is the injection on top of the skin? Will my skin be all red?"

She sounded more like a prosecutor, questioning me for a deposition in a malpractice case, than a patient. I became increasingly cautious in my answers and kept repeating that in plastic surgery, there are never any guarantees. When I told her that the effects of the injections could last for up to a year, she said, "Well, when it wears off in a year, do I come back for another injection?"

By then I knew she was obsessive and refusing to listen to what I was actually saying.

"I have a sense that you're very specific in what you're expecting," I said. "What I'm trying to tell you is that this is not an exact science. Restylane is not going to last a year. It lasts *up* to a year. With some patients, it works for only three to four months. Everybody has a different reaction. I don't want you to come back and be unhappy."

"Okay, what about my lip? See, it's too thin in one corner."

I looked at it carefully. "I could inject Restylane there," I told her, "but it tends not to last as long in the lip."

"Will it make my lip age more quickly?"

"The bottom line," I said, "is that it doesn't age the skin."

"So that has never happened?"

I said no, but by now I knew that I wouldn't inject anything into this woman. She would surely come back complaining, wanting more for free, or claiming malpractice.

"Give me the mirror," she demanded. I handed it to her. There was nothing discernibly wrong with her lip, but she pulled one side more than it should have been pulled and certainly gave it more effect than I ever could with the injection. It also distorted her face. "Will it be like this?"

"No," I said, taking hold of her lip and lifting it the tiniest bit. "It will be like this."

"So, can fat injections make my lip look bigger?"

"You know," I told her, "you really don't have to do anything. You're young, and you're beautiful. Restylane is the only thing I would recommend. I wouldn't recommend fat injections."

"Okay," she said with a melodramatic sigh, and I had the consent form brought in. I handed it to her, and she began reading it aloud. When she came to the part that said Restylane was a hyaluronic acid, she asked me what that meant.

"It's a sugar molecule."

"I've heard that some sugar substitutes are carcinogenic," she said. "Is this carcinogenic?"

That's when I knew I had my out.

"You know, I don't get a clear sense that you really want to do this," I said. "I don't feel comfortable injecting you. I think your expectations don't match what I can deliver."

"No, please," she said as her demeanor changed and her voice became whiny. "I came all the way here, and I need the shot. Is it because I asked too many questions?"

"No. Actually, I like it when patients ask questions. It shows me they're trying to be well informed about their procedures," I explained, trying not to upset her. "But it's clear I can't meet your expectations, so I don't think it is a good idea to try. I'm sorry. There will be no charge for this consultation." I quickly left the room.

Anna wanted a guarantee, and I couldn't give her one. I always say no to guarantees. Furthermore, at the tender age of only twenty-three, her face needed nothing.

As I said, I like patients who ask questions, and I often spend thirty or forty minutes in consultations with new patients. The more they know, the easier the process becomes. But Anna's questions had made it clear that nothing would satisfy her, and that treating her would be risky. Certainly, a woman that is consumed with what she perceives as flaws will become a lifelong plastic surgery patient for another doctor. For me, it simply wasn't worth it. And if I'd had any doubts about my decision, overhearing her conversation with Lorraine as I wrote up her chart in the kitchen dispelled them.

"Why was this consultation free when my first one wasn't?" she asked.

At least ten times.

Finally I heard an exasperated Lorraine say, "There's no charge. There's no discussion. We're finished."

Another patient was a woman in her fifties. She came in for three consultations, wanting a rhinoplasty. Each time, she would push up the tip of her nose and say, "I want something like this."

I tried to explain to her that I couldn't do exactly what she wanted, but she didn't seem to be listening. Then she'd show me a photograph from a magazine and say, "Can you do this?"

On her, I couldn't. The result I can achieve is related to a patient's bone structure and skin elasticity. You can't just have any nose you want. Finally, at the conclusion of our third meeting, I again said that I could not give her the nose she wanted and that I thought she should go elsewhere.

I'm sure she did, and I'm sure she got a nose she wasn't happy with.

People like her go from doctor to doctor until they get someone to do the surgery. Unfortunately, they then go again from doctor to doctor trying to correct mistakes, or still trying to get what wasn't possible in the first place.

Another patient who was determined to get what he wanted came in to talk about his chin. He had a chin like Jay Leno—*plus*. So when he asked if I could augment his chin, I nearly fell off my chair.

"Well," I said, "you already have a pretty prominent chin. Have you had any surgery on it?"

"No, I've never had surgery," he said. But he had to be lying. He definitely did not have a natural chin.

"You haven't had *any* procedures?" I asked.

"I had some injections," he said.

I asked him a few more questions, and it turned out that he had been injected with collagen mixed with tiny ceramic spheres, a substance that is not legal in America. In fact, it had just been taken off the market in Europe. The collagen breaks down and the ceramic remains, and patients often have adverse reactions.

It was obvious that the last thing this man needed was a chin augmentation; there was no way I could make his chin bigger. But he'd come prepared. He pulled out a catalog from his briefcase and showed me the different chin implants that appealed to him.

I felt bad that I couldn't help him. But if someone comes to me for surgery, one of my unwritten contracts is that I decide what is best for the patient.

I decided it was best not to treat him.

"In my opinion, I don't think you would benefit from a chin augmentation," I said. "Your chin projection is already good."

"Are you sure you can't do this?" He looked at me, so earnest, so calm.

"I don't think this is a reasonable operation for you," I said as I stood up and offered my hand. He looked defeated, shook my hand, and left.

There are people I only partially reject, because if they meet certain conditions, I can then help them. When I consult with people who are obese, I have to tell them that they're not yet good candidates for plastic surgery. Not long ago I met with a woman named Felicia, who came in wanting liposuction or a tummy tuck. She said she was in good health, although she added that she took Prozac and smoked a pack of cigarettes a day.

"How much do you weigh?" I asked.

"I'm not sure," she said. "I haven't weighed myself in a while. I bet I weigh about one eighty."

She looked much heavier than that, but she was still in her clothes, so I didn't say anything. I proceeded to tell her what a tummy tuck entailed. I'd make an incision stretching across her body, just above the pubic hair, then remove excess skin and fat and tighten the muscle underneath so that the stomach becomes flat.

"Sometimes, if the skin has good enough elasticity, liposuction will suffice," I told her. "The bottom line is, I have to take a look." She wasn't yet in a gown, so I left the room to give her a chance to change. When I went back in she was holding the gown tight against her body.

"Can you tell I'm a little nervous?" she said.

"I don't blame you," I said with a smile. "This will only take a minute. Now, relax your belly."

"I have no elasticity there."

"You do have stretch marks."

"I gained a lot when I was pregnant. I used to be skinny."

"Liposuction won't do it," I said as I examined the folds of her skin. "You depend on the skin to contract in liposuction. After pregnancies, it's usually either do nothing, or do a tummy tuck."

Next came the hard part.

"The other thing I recommend is, you will get a much better result if you lose weight. If you can lose twenty pounds, not only will you decrease your risk with anesthesia, but I can remove more skin and give you a flatter belly. I know how hard it is to lose weight, because I just lost ten pounds. I recommend you lose at least twenty or thirty pounds and come back in six months. And, to make it even more diffi-cult, you have to try to stop smoking, because you will heal better if you do."

That definitely was not what she wanted to hear.

"I was thinking I would have it done by my daughter's wedding in August," she said.

"I'm afraid not," I said. "My job is to make sure I don't hurt a patient, and that takes precedence over everything else. But I hope I gave you some incentive."

Sometimes I'm saying no to an entirely different kind of request, which always throws me completely off balance. I had done a breast augmentation on a woman named Sophie. She was back for her regular checkup, six months after surgery. She was very pleasant, very pretty. She came by herself, and I had no idea what she did for a living.

As I examined Sophie's breasts to check how they'd healed, one of my staff members was in the room, as always.

"Doctor," Sophie said, looking straight at me, "I love my new sex toys."

What could I say? I kept it simple. "I'm glad."

Another time, I was in an examining room with a patient a day after her surgery.

"I had a dream about you last night," she said.

"That's nice," I said, taking off bandages and making sure that fluid was draining correctly.

"Oh, my God, it was such a dream," she said.

"It was probably the medication," I said.

"There were handcuffs, and leashes, and collars." She looked expectantly at me.

What could I say? So I just laughed.

"Who was wearing the collar?" I asked, pulling off my gloves and quickly leaving the room.

At least she was up-front about her desires. I'd much rather deal with a patient like her than a plastic surgery junkie.

Plastic surgery junkies are impossible to please.

When does a patient cross the line from wanting improvement to obsessively craving it?

I'd say having a surgical procedure every year or two is going too far.

Having multiple breast enlargements. Having multiple rhinoplasties.

Having liposuction on every part of the body that can be liposuctioned. Having a face-lift every few years.

Abuse of injectibles is just as bad. Lots of people want too much Botox, too much Restylane, too much collagen, too much of everything. Their lips become so large it looks as if they were stung by a mutant wasp. They go back for more before they need to. They visit multiple doctors and lie about it. For them, once they see positive results, they become convinced that every other perceived flaw, large or small, real or imagined, must be fixed. And fixed immediately.

One patient kept dropping by the office and saying, "I think I look jowly. Don't I need a face-lift?" We would tell her no, that she looked beautiful, that she should come back in three or four years. Then Lorraine ran into her on the street one day, and she said that she'd been going to her dermatologist for collagen injections to smooth out the lines on her face. Lines, I must say, that only she could see.

She'd crossed the line from looking natural to looking freakishly overdone.

Trust me, I'll get to the freakishly overdone and other mistakes soon. I don't, however, consider patients in their forties and fifties, who've already had several procedures, to be junkies. They are simply exquisitely aware of their bodies. Surgery makes them happier with their lives. Whether it does more for them than a different partner, a different job, or therapy would, I have no idea.

As I said, I'm not the one to judge.

Dorothy, for instance, has been coming to me for years. She is fifty-three and single, and has had a great deal of work done. But I don't think of her as a junkie. She's rational about her needs and expectations.

Dorothy first came to me ten years ago to have a scar corrected on the tip of her nose, a painful reminder of a botched rhinoplasty she'd had a few years before that. Her doctor had made her nose turn up, giving it a perky look that didn't suit her face or her personality.

We hit it off from the very beginning. She told me she was comfortable with me, which surprised her. Most doctors, she said, scared her, and she didn't trust any of them. After several years had passed, she came to talk about her face, particularly her neck, which was starting to go south a little bit. I did her face-lift, which took care of her neck; her eyes; and her nose, trying to return it to the shape it used to have, although it will always be smaller than it was before her first surgery.

Several years later, she was back for a tummy tuck. She explained that even when she was at her skinniest, she'd always had extra flesh on her stomach, which drove her crazy. (Patients with specific complaints like Dorothy's are usually the best candidates for surgery. They have a specific flaw that can't be corrected by either diet or exercise.) She came through the tummy tuck with barely a bruise; she's a very careful patient who pays attention to all pre- and postsurgical instructions.

I still see her regularly for Botox injections. All her surgery, she tells me, was worth every bit of time, money, and pain, as she is now thrilled with her face and body.

"I feel like I've been born again, only better," she said.

It's nice to have such a satisfied patient. Dorothy loves to chat about her boyfriends. Her latest catch is only twenty-six and has no idea how old she is.

"If he knew," she said, "it would probably send him into cardiac arrest."

Dorothy is a perfect example of how having multiple surgeries over ten to fifteen years can be okay.

One nurse I know has had five surgeries over fifteen years: a breast reduction, a rhinoplasty, an upper eyelid–lift, a laser of the lower lids, liposuction, and fat injections. Now that she's approaching fifty, she's thinking of a face-lift. I think that's within reason.

Another patient, Leigh, originally came to me for a tummy tuck after losing thirty pounds, and she had drooping, excess skin. But this also stemmed from her body type. She'd always hated her stomach, telling me it was like a "pouch" even when she was at her thinnest. In fact, the more weight she lost, the more her stomach pouched out. It was just the way she was built.

Leigh was delighted after surgery. She told me she never realized what a big difference it would make to have a brand-new belly, and she couldn't wait to run out and buy a bikini. So delighted was she, actually, that she came back for a face-lift, a brow-lift, and a breast-lift. Again, she was delighted by her newfound ability to wear low-cut dresses and show off her cleavage.

She often comes in for Botox and Restylane, which help diminish the angry little lines between her eyebrows. She's thinking about more surgery, but I told her she's not ready yet. When she is ready for another face-lift, perhaps in ten years or so, I'll do it.

If she's not, I won't.

If she goes to another surgeon for a procedure after I recommend that she doesn't, she'll be veering into junkie land.

If she doesn't, she'll just be a satisfied patient.

And that is the best kind of patient.

Eight

CELEBRITY CATASTROPHES AND OTHER HORRIBLE MISTAKES I HAVE SEEN

HOW CAN YOU TELL WHEN A CELEBRITY HAS HAD PLASTIC SURGERY?

When he or she denies it.

Okay, that may be a bit too flippant. But it always makes me laugh when a superstar goes on and on about her yoga, and her homeopathy, and her workout routine, and her Ayurvedic face oils, and all her other "beauty secrets," when in truth her beauty secret is the plastic surgeon she sees on a regular basis for every conceivable injectible coupled with as much surgery as she can stand.

Actually, I feel sorry for celebrities when it comes to maintaining their looks. As Hollywood standards of beauty have become more and more ludicrous—the ultrathin yet sublimely toned body, complete with large, perky breasts and a perfectly shaped derriere, faces devoid of any lines of character and humor—the need to appear young and perfect becomes not a luxury but a necessity for actors and actresses trying to stay in the game. As it stands, they don't have a lot of choice in the matter. Their faces and bodies are their livelihood. If they choose to be actresses, they know they will be exposing themselves forevermore to the merciless gaze of public scrutiny, which damns them for getting older yet mocks them for wanting to look younger and better.

It's either be Botoxed/starved/plucked/manicured/sliced to within an inch of your life, or throw in the towel and move back to Topeka.

If you don't believe me, check out www.awfulplasticsurgery.com and see for yourself.

So celebrities flock to plastic surgeons. And pretend they don't.

Well, a few can't pretend. Actress Jennifer Grey, who was so adorable in the 1987 film *Dirty Dancing*, had a distinctive nose. She had it bobbed. It was a terrific nose job. But the problem for Jennifer is that having a terrific nose isn't the same as having a *distinctive* nose. As she has admitted, she literally became unrecognizable. No one believed she was the same adorable actress from *Dirty Dancing*. And there was nothing Jennifer could do to replace her lost nose.

Perhaps, someday, a celebrated superstar will finally come out of the closet and say, "Yes, I want to look as good as I possibly can, and I'm going to do whatever I can to maintain my beauty, which the industry forces me to maintain if I want to be able to work and have a career that doesn't die when I hit the age of forty, and here's the name of my plastic surgeon, and I'm proud of it." Then the stigma will lessen and the snarky comments will stop.

But this isn't going to happen anytime soon.

You'd think that celebrities, who have money and can pick and choose from the world's best plastic surgeons, would avail themselves of the very best. But no. I find it shocking how much terrible work is done on these famous faces. Too often, instead of looking natural, they overdo it, becoming caricatures of their former selves.

I can let you in on a few trade secrets. Trained eyes can instantly spot the telltale signs of surgical procedures, especially when things go wrong. Even untrained eyes can easily pick up on asymmetry. If you think a face is somehow "off," it probably is.

From top to bottom:

- Hairline: A hairline that is too high is a dead giveaway, as are sideburns that start up too high. Excessive pulling of the skin during a face-lift or brow-lift gives that result.
- Face-lift: The face is pulled so tight you can practically bounce quarters off the cheekbones. An overly aggressive face-lift takes away too much skin, so the face looks pulled, stretched, or shiny. The person can also look unnatural, unlike his or her old self. There is no animation at the corner of the mouth. If earlobes are hanging way down, or if there are wide scars near the ears, that's a telltale giveaway too.

  If the skin is pulled too tightly under the chin, we have a nickname for that: popsicle on a stick.
- Brow: Brows are smooth and shiny, wrinkle-free. It's just not natural. Every adult has wrinkles. They give you character. A brow frozen by Botox has no wrinkles and no expression. When you talk, you can look like a zombie.
- Upper eye: Botched eyelid surgery leaves people unable to close their eyes, because too much skin has been taken out of their lids. Eyes can also appear sunken, making a person look like a cadaver. Sometimes people have that deer-in-the-headlights look, or the eyes are unnaturally open, so they seem to be staring. Or the natural animation in the eyes is gone.
- Lower eyelid: If it is pulled down, surgery was done incorrectly, or if too much white of the eye is visible, something went wrong. It's a bloodhound look, attractive only on bloodhounds. Sometimes, a mistake leaves the lower eye bowed rather than straight across, or too sloped and high in the corners.
- Cheeks: Cheek implants placed in the wrong plane can injure the nerves, leaving people looking as if they had a stroke. Implants can also stick out at unnatural angles, making a person look like a mannequin. I've also seen implants placed too close to the midline, and the person ends up looking like she has walnuts in her cheeks.
- Nose: If the nose appears to be too small, too turned up, too

pinched in, too thin, or too chiseled, then you know that too much cartilage was taken out. It is unfortunately way too easy to slim a nose down too much. The top can be pinched and turned up, making it unnaturally perky. Or the cartilage at the top can collapse.

The biggest giveaway: You can look right into the nostrils.

- Nasolabial fold: If you see absolutely no nasolabial folds, the lines that run from the mouth to the nose, there is something wrong. Even my kids have them, although of course they are very, very slight.

- Lips: If the lips are immobile, or if they look like they have a brick in them, some kind of implant has been inserted. Lips with implants don't seem to move when the person talks, or they are so puffy and disproportionately large for the face that they practically hit the tip of the nose.

- Chin: Sometimes a chin is too pointed, created by putting in a tiny little implant. That problem is becoming less common because the new implants wrap around the inside of the chin and give it a more natural look.

- Jaw: A perfectly clean jawline is an instant giveaway. Jaws with perfect angles are simply not natural after a certain age. Bad face-lifts give, as I said above, that popsicle-on-a-stick look: a thin neck and a head that appears to be hanging off of it.

- Neck: A neck can look scooped from overaggressive liposuction during a face-lift, when so much fat is removed that there's nothing left between the muscles and the skin. Normally, skin moves with the muscle underneath. If too much fat is taken out, resulting in skin directly over muscle, then every little movement of the muscle becomes too obvious and strange looking.

- Breasts: Breasts should not bob up around the shoulders, nearly grazing the chin. They also should not look like unnatural, immobile spheres. And they won't if they're the correct size and put under the muscle.

I don't do pectoral implants for men, either. The contour is too artificial. If pecs look like grapefruits on the chest instead of having a natural flowing curvature, blame it on implants.

- Buttocks: The buttocks have a bizarre new shape. I even heard about somebody who used breast implants in a woman's butt. A butt is not a breast. You sit on it, lie down on it. Your gluteus maximus is the largest muscle group in your body. It's ridiculous to put a foreign body in an area that is tension bearing.

  In fact, it's more than ridiculous. It's insane.

  Buttocks can also get a funny, indented, unnatural look from too much liposuction. You have to be very careful—if you scoop out too much, the butt can end up looking flat and shapeless.

- Thighs: Liposuction can cause rippled skin and indentations. It can also worsen preexisting cellulite.

Joan Rivers has become the poster child for excessive surgery, which is why so many of my patients beg me not to make them look like her. She doesn't look natural. When she smiles, her face doesn't move. If you look closely, you can see that the skin on her jaw is puckered. And she's one of the few celebrities who are up-front about their many operations. I guess she has to be, because the results are so glaringly obvious.

I've had a chance to look at some famous faces up close, some in person, some in pictures. Here's what my practiced eye tells me about these celebrities:

Paul McCartney, to me, is a familiar face that has changed irreparably. Instead of looking forever young, he looks forever startled.

Not long ago, my wife and I ran into a well-known singer, whose talent I respect tremendously. I'd met him before at a baseball game, so I reintroduced myself, and we had a nice chat for a few minutes, long enough for me to notice that there was a glaring flaw in his face. His earlobes were noticeably pulled down, which happens when the skin is sewn back badly, under tension, after a face-lift.

Former *Cosmopolitan* editor Helen Gurley Brown is, in my opinion, an example of an overdone face-lift. Her face has been so strongly pulled that her eyes become slanted and her brows seem to have moved halfway up her forehead. That's a consequence of an overdone eyebrow-lift, which changes the natural shape of the eyebrow and the aperture of the eye.

Meg Ryan exhibits a different problem. She suddenly appeared one day with visibly altered lips. I'd say she had Gore-Tex put in her lips. You can tell because her face is smiling while her lips remain immobile.

Barbra Streisand had a face-lift but did not have her eyes done, and they look out of sync.

Marie Osmond looks like a wax dummy. The middle of her face looks weird, as if she has had too many injectibles, and her eyebrows arc unnaturally.

Burt Reynolds looks like he has had a face-lift and a nose job. Actually, they don't look bad. But his face looks like it has two parts now. The lower face is a forty-five-year-old man, while his eyes look like those of an old man. I would have done laser around the eyes, or some Botox. It's always best to have all the parts of your face appear to be the same age. If you address only half of your face, you end up looking weird.

David Gest, who was briefly married to Liza Minnelli, had a bad brow-lift. It was pulled up way too high. Like Paul McCartney, he looks perpetually surprised.

Sharon Stone is an example of too much Botox, injected badly. Proper application is based on a strong knowledge of anatomy. If you totally deactivate the forehead, the result is a mask, not a mobile, expressive face.

I could go on, but you need only open the pages of any weekly celebrity-oriented magazine to see the damage done to the rich and famous.

Celebrities, of course, are not the only people who have had bad plastic surgery. Waking up to find terrible results—that they'll look artificial, or too obviously "done"—is the most common worry for all my patients.

And frankly, they should worry. Cosmetic surgery is all about judgment. In a single surgery there are dozens of important judgment calls, moments where if the surgeon turns to the right instead of the left, the

result will be quite different. There are hundreds of excellent plastic surgeons in this country, but there are also plenty of doctors who are doing
things I wouldn't do and that I consider to be mistakes.

I'm not saying I have never made a mistake. But I'm cautious by nature
in my work, and I don't push things. It's always better to go back and do
more, rather than make a drastic change that can't ever be fixed.

It's vitally important for people to understand that plastic surgery is a
serious business. While the vast majority of cases turn out just fine,
some do not. It's critical to be cautious. Death from plastic surgery is
rare, but it does happen. Mistakes in judgment, however, are not rare.

For one thing, there can be endless mistakes during surgery itself.
Some of them are absurd, like the five thousand cases a year of things
such as sponges and instruments left inside patients. When I do surgery,
we count and count and count. I look three and four times; you have to
be compulsive.

But those aren't the mistakes that show. The mistakes that do show are
usually cases where doctors aren't careful or well trained enough, or, sad
to say, where their desire to make money overwhelms their judgment
and prompts them to cut corners. Or allows them to be willing to please
their patients, even when their patients demand something that is
absolutely not suitable.

Every day patients come to me in despair. Wanting the implants taken
out of their lumpy, misshapen lips. Wanting their breasts to look realistic. Wanting to go back to their original faces. Unfortunately, that can
rarely happen.

I'm always happy to get new patients. But I prefer getting them the
first time around rather than when they need a botched procedure fixed.

I CAN'T BE MR. FIX-IT IF
- too much skin has been removed. During a face-lift. During a
  tummy tuck. During a nose job. During an eye job. Less is more.
  I can always go back and take more out. I can't put more in.
- a motor nerve has been cut during a face-lift, paralyzing that area
  of the face.

- incisions have been made in the wrong place. In a face-lift, for instance, if the incisions are too far forward, in front of the ear, there is no way to correct them. All you can do is wait a number of years until the skin has sagged and can handle another face-lift. Only then can the scar be put in the right place.
- body parts are moved to the wrong place. In a breast reduction, for example, if the nipple is moved too high, it is impossible to correct.

One of the worst cases I ever saw was clearly malpractice—the woman's thigh-lift had been done so poorly that her labial lips were permanently pulled apart, and her vagina was grotesquely swollen, red, and irritated. She needed skin grafts, which would result in additional scarring to ease her pain and mutilation. I don't slam other doctors, though. Unless I was in the operating room, I'll never know their side of the story.

But I can often make a pretty good guess.

Here are lots more details about some of the disasters I see.

Eyelids

One of the most common disasters I see is botched eyelids, where patients can't close their eyes after surgery. One of the reasons is that far too many unqualified doctors are doing this procedure. A doctor who is licensed to do surgery can do any kind of surgery. That's not to say that plastic surgeons never get bad results, or that eye doctors and dermatologists never get good ones. But there are doctors who decide they're perfectly able to take out fat in the upper and lower eyelid after only a weekend seminar. The lectures can make it seem like a benign, relatively simple operation—but it's not. Muscle injury is a risk. You need to pull the fat out of the eye very carefully and thoughtfully, because if you make even the slightest mistake and injure the muscle by cutting it, it's possible that the patient will not be able to fully open the eye afterward. Using an eye lubricant is mandatory until the problem can be resolved. If it can't be resolved, you'll be using lubricant forever. You might also end up with double vision.

Eyelid surgery is tricky. If you take out too little fat, you don't get a satisfying result. If you take out too much, you create a gaunt look. I admit that I push the envelope more than some doctors; I take out more skin and fat than I did when I first started out fifteen years ago. I've honed my technique after doing thousands of these operations over the years. That's why someone who has just taken a weekend seminar about how to do this procedure is more likely to make mistakes.

Jack had gone to a doctor for what should have been a complication-free procedure to remove fat and excess skin on his lower eyelids. But the surgery was a disaster—too much skin was taken out from under his eyes and left his lower lids drooping. Jack suddenly looked older than his thirty-eight years, not younger, and also a bit strange. He underwent several surgeries in an attempt to correct the problem, and none of them worked.

By the time Jack came to see me, after being referred by his eye doctor, he was very depressed and discouraged. His eyelids were destroyed, and his eyes were continually dry and irritated. I explained that he needed more skin under the eyelid to correct the problem. It's not possible to do skin grafts in that area, but I could do a face-lift. That would allow me to move skin up from another part of his face.

It was a very difficult case. I did an endoscopic face-lift, making an incision in his temple and mouth. I elevated all of the tissue and separated it from the bone. By shifting the skin toward his eyes, I provided the excess tissue he needed. Then an ocular plastic surgeon took over when it was time to work around the eyes.

Jack looks like a human being now. He told me I changed his life and made him normal again.

I wish I could say the same for John. I didn't work on him, but I heard about his case. He was in surgery to have the puffiness removed from his upper and lower eyes. While under sedation, he began moving a little bit. The anesthesiologist was giving him medication to help him sleep more deeply, but he didn't do it in time. The surgeon, who was cutting out the fat in his upper lid, must have cut into a place he shouldn't have.

At first, no one knew that anything was wrong. But when John woke up, he couldn't see. His private duty nurse called the resident when she couldn't find the doctor who'd done the surgery. The resident freaked out and immediately called in several ophthalmologists. They assumed that John had a hematoma, a pooling of blood under the skin, and took appropriate steps to get rid of the blood, but John still could not see. That led them to assume that there must be bleeding behind the eye. On examination, they saw that his bleeding was *in* the eye.

Over the next few weeks, John regained some of his vision, but he still couldn't see perfectly. He also started developing a posttraumatic cataract, which must be treated or he could become permanently blind in that eye. Undoubtedly, this case will end up in court. It's every patient's worst nightmare when it comes to eye surgery. Going in to remove puffiness should not result in removing your vision!

Breasts, or the Double Bubble

When I first met Ashley I couldn't help noticing what a beautiful woman she was at the age of thirty-seven. She'd had her breasts augmented by a surgeon near her home in Queens, and there had been a problem. I asked her to take off her gown, and I looked at her breasts.

There was a problem, all right.

About five years earlier, she had had a transumbilical breast augmentation. In this procedure, a long tube is put through the belly button, and the implant is placed through it. Women are attracted to this method because there are no incisions made on the breasts and therefore no scars. The limitation of this technique is that it only allows placement of the implant above the muscle.

What doctors don't tell patients is that the implant, over time, can move and change shape. The implant is in one place, usually sitting too high, and the breast is in another. This creates a distorted chest. We call it the double bubble. The only person the double bubble is good for is *me*. It starts a whole cycle of corrective surgery for its unfortunate victims. Fixing this double bubble is the most common secondary surgery that I do.

Ashley's implant looked like a rock sitting up there. She was miserably self-conscious about it, and I didn't blame her. Fixing it would not be easy, because you have to adjust two opposites; you're trying to increase one thing and decrease something else. First, you remove the old implant, and then you put a new implant under the muscle, where it really belongs, and at the same time you do a breast-lift.

It's not that doctors don't know how to do it right the first time. They're just misleading people, trying to get business by advertising a quick and scar-free procedure. If you put the implant in *over* the muscle, you can do it quickly, using local anesthetic in an office. If you do it right, under the muscle, it's a longer operation, with more postoperative pain.

But if you do it right the first time, you won't end up with a double bubble.

I'm also treating a woman who has desperately been trying to correct a mistake made during her breast-lift surgery. Her surgeon apparently measured wrong and made the nipple too high on the breast. This woman has already had two surgeries trying to correct it, and she remains unhappy, with good reason. The implant is still too low, and the nipple is still too high. I operated on her, putting in a larger implant, and I was then able to move the nipple down somewhat. I couldn't move it down to the ideal position, because that would have produced an unattractive scar. She looks better, but not perfect. It was frustrating for us both, because I like things to be perfect. But not everything can be fixed. And now she's stuck with a distorted breast for the rest of her life.

Cheek Implants

"This one bothers me," said Belinda, pointing to her left cheek. An attractive woman of fifty-five, she'd had a face-lift and cheek implants nine months before. "It seems to get in the way of my lip. The other one is just fine. I like my doctor, but when he said, 'Oh, it's only a millimeter off,' I didn't think that was right. Even my hairdresser noticed that there was something off, without my having said a word about it."

I felt around her cheek. The implants were made of Gore-Tex, which is soft, the same material used in jackets.

"It's a good implant," I said, "but a little difficult to remove."

"Well, should I have him try to move it up?" she asked. "How difficult is that? Or should I just have him take it out?"

"Those are the choices you have," I said. "Let me take a better look."

I put on gloves and moved my fingers around in her mouth for a minute or so, then stood back.

"Smile for me, please," I said. "When you smile, does it feel constricting?"

"Yes."

"Does it hurt you?"

"It's a little uncomfortable."

"Is it constant discomfort, or just when you smile?"

"I always notice it. The other one, I don't notice at all. I feel like this left one is encroaching on my lip."

"That's because it's too low, and it's a little bit mobile. I can feel the edge of it from the inside. It's a tough question of what to do, but I will give you my opinion. It's a matter of how much discomfort you have. That's the bottom line. Having done a number of cheek implants, the one lesson I have learned is that if it's not in the right position, it's almost impossible to take the same implant and try to reposition it. I've tried that."

I get a fair amount of referrals for secondary cheek implants because I wrote a paper about it in 1995 with Sherrell Aston and Ed Ivy for a journal called *Plastic and Reconstructive Surgery* titled "Malar Augmentation with Silicone Implants." If the pocket created from the cheek to hold the implant is in the wrong place, I have to take the implant out and make another pocket in the right place. It's very difficult to do it so that the implant doesn't slip from the new pocket to the old pocket. Which meant Belinda would have to have the old implant taken out, let her cheek heal, and then get a new one. I told her that.

"It's more complex, but I take them out, wait six months, and then if you choose, I go back and put the implant in. By then, everything is healed and closed up. I'm afraid that by going in and trying to reposition, there is a very significant chance that the implant will slip."

Then came the clincher.

"The thing is," Belinda said, "I didn't really go in for cheek implants. I went in for my eyes and I ended up with more. Which is okay," she hastened to add. I don't know why she was giving her surgeon the benefit of the doubt when he'd clearly screwed up, but many patients are like that. They don't want to believe their trust has been badly misplaced. "His explanation for me needing cheek implants was that whenever you do something underneath the eye, you need to lift up the cheek, to give it definition. He said there was a lack of cheek structure. So now I'm wondering what it will look like if I take them out."

"I don't think it will make much of a difference, really, because they're small implants," I said. "What I recommend is taking them out. For all I know, you'll come back after your cheek has healed and tell me you're happy with your old cheeks. But if you then decide you could use some prominence, I'll put them back in." I sat back and took off my gloves. "I would also recommend going back to your surgeon and talking about it," I added. "I think the best policy is to be open."

She seemed somewhat reluctant to do that.

"The only thing that bothered me—and I like this doctor—is that he said that this implant *did* look like it slipped. But then he said, 'I think it was fine when I did it. How did it feel when it was first in?' I told him I didn't know, it was swollen. And it concerned me that he said it was off by at most one millimeter. That's why I felt I needed another opinion."

"Just go back to him and be very, very open with him."

I could have crucified that guy for his sloppy work and cavalier attitude, but I also knew his ego would take the biggest hit when Belinda told him that she came to see me. He had put her implants in the wrong pocket, plus the pocket he made was too big. He was full of it when he claimed the implant was only one millimeter off.

It was completely in the wrong place.

Of course, it wouldn't be appropriate for me to tell Belinda how her doctor screwed up and encourage her to take out the implants and fix her up. First of all, if she goes back to him, he'll have to do it without charge. Why should she have to pay me to correct his mistake when he is perfectly capable of taking them out? It's really hard to botch such an easy procedure.

What infuriated me the most was how this doctor took advantage of Belinda. She hadn't needed cheek implants at all. Her doctor was greedy, plain and simple. He convinced a vulnerable patient that she needed an unnecessary procedure, and now she has to deal with a complication from something she didn't need or want in the first place. It's a disgrace.

Luckily for Belinda, her incompetent surgeon didn't do worse. He could have injured the facial nerves that allow you to animate your face. Then she would have looked like she'd had a stroke.

Cheek Reduction

One fad that almost always has negative consequences is the removal of the buccal fat pads. Doctors remove pockets of fat above the molar in each cheek.

This used to be a common procedure for teenagers, as it gave them the appearance of having high cheekbones. That's fine while you're young, but as you age, your cheeks will start to look sunken in and haggard. You'll wish you'd retained those pads, but there is no way to put them back in.

People have come to see me ten years after having had the procedure. They're devastated when they hear the bad news. Faces tend to thin out naturally as we age, and the most attractive face is full, because that conveys youthfulness.

Liposuction

Liposuction can't remove cellulite. Period.

If your doctor tells you liposuction can remove cellulite, run out the door and never look back! I see plenty of people with horribly rippled skin as a result of unnecessary liposuction. Their legs and buttocks may also be misshapen or uneven. When that happens, all I can do to fix it is perform a thigh-lift, which is not a surgery I'm fond of. You redrape the skin, which is good, but then you have a long scar that really does show. You can also inject fat to fix that problem a little, but it doesn't totally solve it. It is much smarter to do just a little reduction, which gives just a little enhancement, than to take these big leaps. One young woman who came to me had had too much liposuction done on her belly, and it caused all these ripples on her abdomen. Terrible. I had to put fat back in. It probably happened because the doctor who did liposuction on her used a cannula that was too large. That was definitely malpractice.

Liposuction is one of the areas of plastic surgery where mistakes in judgment can lead not only to rippled skin but also to death. Take out too much fat and fluid, and the patient can go into shock and cardiac arrest. There are doctors who take out ten to twenty quarts, which is ridiculous and shouldn't be done. In any liposuction, you lose some blood, and in a massive liposuction, you can lose quite a bit. Up to a third of the material that comes out during liposuction is blood. During the procedure, we inject fluid to compensate, to keep the body in balance, and that has to be done carefully and cautiously. Adding the fluid can overdilute the blood and lessen its ability to carry oxygen. In medical terms, liposuction is basically an exercise in hemodynamics (blood circulation).

When deaths happen during liposuction, they may be the result of massive amounts of fat being taken out. According to guidelines that we have at NYU, which I was involved in writing, any patient who is having more than five quarts taken out during liposuction should have the work done in the hospital. And frankly, I think it should be done infrequently, if at all. There's a physician in New York who proposes massive liposuction on obese patients, and I think that's asking for trouble. Eventually it will cause a death.

Liposuction just should not be thought of as a substitute for sensible weight reduction. It's crucial to turn down the seriously overweight patient, who is likely to suffer complications during surgery. To say nothing of not addressing the issues that caused the patient to be overweight in the first place. Liposuction removes fat cells in specific areas. If a patient needs more than ten pounds taken out in a "problem area," I won't do it. It's not safe.

Lose the weight and come back to see me. Then I'll be happy to take care of you.

Lasers

There are lots of different lasers used to resurface the skin—Erbium, for instance, is less penetrating, and CO_2 is more penetrating. When women with dark or olive-toned complexions have chemical peels or laser treatments for wrinkle reduction, there is a very high probability that the pigment of their skin will be changed. It might go lighter, or it might go darker. Then she is cursed with different colors of skin, a mistake that can never be repaired.

A woman from Morocco came to see me with this exact problem. Due to hormonal changes, the skin under her eyes had darkened. After a botched peel, she now had two-tone skin.

"I think you should start with a bleaching cream," I told her. "The standard one is four percent, twice a day every day. Use it for six to eight weeks, and when you come back to New York, if that doesn't work, I have a pharmacist who'll make you a six percent bleaching cream."

"Is it going to be better?" She was young and attractive, and understandably distressed.

"It won't be completely better, but it will definitely be better," I had to tell her. "Someone with your skin tone is unfortunately more prone to these pigment changes. I wouldn't suggest using a laser for darker-skin-toned patients, or any kind of peels whatsoever. If it can potentially do more harm for only a slight improvement, the treatment doesn't make sense. It isn't worth the risk."

If she wasn't satisfied with the result of the bleaching, there wouldn't be much I could do. When skin is damaged with laser, it is possible to fix with skin grafts, but that is extreme and difficult to accomplish.

Noses

People ask me when they'll see the final result of their rhinoplasty.

I tell them, "When you die."

You might not see the final outcome of a rhinoplasty for years, because the nose keeps changing. The contraction of the scar continues for years. That argues for great caution during any nose procedure.

Decades ago, plastic surgeons were very aggressive with rhinoplasty, taking out a lot of cartilage and bone. But it's difficult to replace cartilage and bone once they are taken out.

Of course, nose jobs used to be much more common and much more popular. Now it is the fifth most popular surgical procedure, far eclipsed by face-lifts and liposuction. Still, there are some famously bad noses. You need only look at the puny, collapsing remnant of Michael Jackson's nose to see how far a surgeon can go in destroying bone and tissue. Taking out too much is the most common mistake in nose work, and it gives that telltale pinched and turned-up look.

I do far fewer noses than I used to do, and patients nearly always ask to keep their ethnicity intact, which wasn't something you used to hear. Recently a very pretty woman in her late twenties came to see me. She had an overly long, projecting nose, and although she'd been wanting to have it done for years, she'd been reluctant out of fear that she would have an obviously "done" nose. She didn't hesitate to have me do a breast-lift for her—she felt it was necessary after having had two children—but she scheduled the nose surgery and then canceled, and then scheduled it again. Finally she had the nerve to go through with it. I maintained a little bit of the curvature of the nose, keeping the shape but making it smaller. She was happy with the result.

There are fewer rhinoplasties as people decide that it is okay to have an ethnic nose, or to have one with distinctive imperfections. When I was a teenager, it seemed that every seventeen-year-old girl I knew on Long Island had her nose done. Times have changed, and I think that's great. I don't even do young teenagers' noses. Starting at age seventeen, I'm willing to consider it.

Face-Lifts

Julie came to me years ago, referred by a doctor I know. She was a very pretty woman in her fifties, and she wanted her face, eyes, and brow done. We had a nice chat and Lorraine gave her the estimate, and then I never heard from her again. That happens.

Out of the blue, at six-thirty one evening, just when I was getting ready to go home, I heard a woman's voice over the outside intercom, crying hysterically that she'd been mutilated and begging to see me. It was Julie. She explained that she'd gone to see someone highly recommended by her friends, and he was supposed to do an endoscopic brow-lift, which requires only a small incision. But then when she was already under, he gave her a huge incision across her head. She had long, thin, blond hair, and she had lost a lot of hair along her scalp from ear to ear. In addition, her surgeon had pulled her skin too tight, and she looked like a cat lady.

That night, I did a lot of hand-holding. But at that point, there was nothing I could do to help her. She was fresh off the surgery, with a weird look to her. Eventually it would soften up and look a little bit better, but nothing could be done about the fact that the scars were placed inappropriately.

Botched face-lifts are usually next to impossible to repair. When too much skin is taken out, you have to wait years for it to relax and return to a more normal look. If the redraping of the skin was done incorrectly, it is possible to go back in, open up the skin, and redrape it properly. The pull is usually at forty five degrees. If it is done wrong, the cheeks will look bunched up.

If scars are really bad, they may be able to be fixed when the skin relaxes—this can take years—and there is some laxity that makes another procedure possible. If too much fat is taken out, you can use fat grafts to plump up the skin a bit.

Body-Lifts

I've known Tanya, a massage therapist, for years, since she first came to me after losing 160 pounds. She did it the hard way, cutting down on calories and carbohydrates and exercising for at least an hour a day.

When she got down to her ideal weight, Tanya wanted information about a lower-body-lift. It involves long incisions on the hips and thighs to eliminate excess skin and fat, and it's a procedure I don't do because it can leave significant scars. I don't think the tradeoff is worth it. But I agreed to do a fair amount of liposuction on her legs and back, and to give her a face-lift.

Although Tanya was pleased with the results, she still wanted the lower-body-lift to get rid of the last bits of excess, droopy skin. She consulted many doctors but no one would do it, because they knew, as I did, that it wouldn't be worth her trouble for minimal results. I didn't hear from her for about eight years, until I ran into her at a seminar I was giving at a salon on the Upper East Side. She told me her story, and it was gruesome.

Eventually she found a surgeon to do a lower-body-lift. It went well. After she healed, she decided that she wanted her breasts to be slightly larger and lifted, and having had a good experience with that doctor, she went back to him. Although she initially thought of having only her breasts done, he convinced her that she should also have some work done on her upper arms.

He proposed enlarging her breasts, and on her arms he performed an operation of his own design, cutting under the arm and pulling up the skin. It was far less invasive than the traditional way of dealing with fat hanging from arms, so it sounded good to Tanya. She hadn't thought that her arms looked that bad, but she trusted him.

That's when she began experiencing problems. Somehow during the surgery, a nerve was injured.

Tanya now has no control over the muscle that holds down the scapula, the two wings in your back. When she lifts her arm, her bone sticks way out, which looks ugly. Worse, she is functionally unable to lift her arm above her shoulder, which is a disaster for a masseuse.

When her arm didn't get better, Tanya called the doctor, and he told her to "hang in," that it would improve. When it didn't, she went to a physical therapist, who suggested that Tanya might have a nerve problem. So she went back to see the doctor, initially with no intention of suing. She just wanted him to fix the problem. Instead of agreeing to help her, he became hostile and went as far as suggesting that she'd had some previous problem that was causing the arm problem.

"I thought my boyfriend was going to punch him," she told me.

She was about to start her malpractice trial against him when I saw her. She said that her expert witness believed that the doctor had cut the nerve, or that he had somehow looped a suture around the nerve and strangled it.

Unless she has extensive physical therapy twice a week, she is in constant, unremitting pain. She was suing the doctor to get money to pay for her physical therapy; the surgery took place in a state where malpractice awards are capped at $250,000, so she has no hope of being compensated for lost income, let alone pain and suffering.

Not long after our conversation at the salon, she came to me to talk about her breasts. She was angry at the doctor, not so much for the mistake he'd made on her arm but for the way he'd flagrantly disregarded what she had wanted done on her breasts. She had asked to become a size C cup and instead he made her an extremely large and disproportionate DD.

It was shocking when I looked at her. First he put in the wrong size implants, and then he hadn't fixed her loose skin, which was her original complaint. She'd wanted only a lift, not implants, and he'd persuaded her to get both. Now her breasts were totally out of sync with her body, so huge they were pulling on her shoulders.

We agreed that I would do breast reduction surgery after her trial. Her bad experience had scared her and made her understandably nervous about more surgery, but she didn't feel she had much choice.

Amazingly, though, after everything she'd endured, Tanya was still positive about plastic surgery. When it worked.

"I'd much rather have a face-lift than a new car," she told me. "I would rather look at myself in the mirror each day and smile because I know I look good."

After all she'd been through, she still thought she might have more work done in the future, perhaps to have her still-saggy thighs fixed. She said the lesson she'd learned was not that plastic surgery was bad, but that research into the best possible surgeons and techniques was crucial.

"Just because a doctor is good at one thing doesn't mean he's going to be good at another," she said with a rueful grin. "This guy who screwed me up sure knew the lower body. He just didn't know anything about the upper body. He should have stopped while he was ahead and not been so greedy."

If more plastic surgeons concentrated on what they did best, I wouldn't be seeing so many mistakes.

Nine

TAKING THE PLUNGE

AGING IS ANNOYING AND FRUSTRATING. FOR PEOPLE WHO WANT TO MIN-
imize its effects, it can also be expensive.

But worth it!

Coming to the decision to have plastic surgery isn't easy, and I don't
encourage people to do it lightly. My job isn't to tell my potential patients
what they should look like, or to suggest procedures, or to talk them into
changing their bodies or faces. In my initial consultations I have a standard speech. You must think about why you're considering doing it. You
must do it only for yourself. And you must understand that any plastic
surgery procedure is real surgery. Admittedly with low risks, but very
real risks nonetheless.

I lay out the possibilities about particular techniques, but I never
encourage anyone to go forward with procedures. The pushiest I get is to
say, "I think it's a reasonable procedure."

I don't believe in the hard-sell philosophy. Having elective surgery
must be entirely your decision. In the worst-case scenario, I could wind
up getting blamed if a procedure isn't entirely satisfactory, or if patients

spend far more than they initially imagined was feasible for whatever they had done.

Naturally, some people listen, and some people don't. Some have thought about making an appointment for months, if not years, before they consult me, and others have come on impulse.

So what pushes people to take the plunge?

For some, one too many overheard and snarkily whispered comments from a "friend" or a relative provides the necessary incentive. Others are tired of looking in the mirror every day and being unhappy with their reflection. In our increasingly ageist society, they justifiably believe that they must look good to keep their jobs. (And not just look good—look *younger*.) Still others see it as proof that they're worthy, while others are more resigned, looking at it as merely an inevitable stage in the aging process. Often, friends have procedures done, look refreshed and younger, and that's reason enough.

However the decision is made, I don't judge my patients. If they want surgery, there's a good chance that the changes will please them. For me, that's a valid choice.

A bit more problematic are those patients who are indecisive. They come in for a consultation, or perhaps *many* consultations, but then they say no. Their no still never really puts the matter to rest. They may have decided against surgery, but every time they walk by a mirror, they can't help lifting up their cheeks thinking about how much better they'd look with a nicely defined jawline and a smooth, uncrepey neck, and eyelids that no longer droop and make them look sleepy or perpetually angry. They'd undoubtedly look much better if they had some work done, but the notion is just too scary.

Scarier than their regrets.

At the end of the day, though, for whatever reasons, I've found that people take the plunge only when they are ready. When the timing is right.

Afterward, some patients practically run down the street, happy to announce to all and sundry on Park Avenue that they've gone under the knife, while others remain totally secretive. One of my favorite stories about the hazards of trying to keep surgery a secret happened about thirteen years ago. Alexandra, a lovely woman in her fifties, a retired editor, came in for a brow-lift and dermabrasion. In those days, before the introduction of endoscopic surgery, a brow-lift necessitated an incision across her entire head, from ear to ear. The scar was pretty fierce. Plus, Alexandra's dermabrasion around her lips made her look burned, and she was covered with a yellowish clear fluid for the first five days. Not surprisingly, she absolutely did not want a single soul to know what she'd done, and certainly not to see her. She sneaked back into her apartment, called the doorman and told him that she was sick and didn't want to be disturbed, and took to her bed.

Being a helpful doorman, he went up to her apartment the next day because she had received a package. He wanted to put it inside her door so it would be there for her convenience. He knocked, got no response, and when he opened the door to her apartment, he heard her TV on and looked toward the bedroom. To his horror, he saw Alexandra spread out on the bed, her head a bloody mess and her face looking like a forest fire. He ran out thinking she was dead and immediately called for help. She, meanwhile, having no idea that he had been there, woke up and went into the bathroom. She was sitting on the toilet with the bathroom door ajar when a half dozen firemen and policemen suddenly kicked the bathroom door fully open to see what was going on.

Luckily for all concerned, Alexandra didn't have a heart attack from the shock. Later, she did manage to laugh about it. "Besides," she told me, "by the time the whole thing was over, everybody in New York City knew what I had done!"

Although that was years ago, when plastic surgery was not as common as it is now, I've found that many of my patients still fall into the secretive category. They hesitate before telling friends or colleagues, or even family members. In some circles, it is still practically considered taboo to have a procedure; in others, almost a pressure to do it.

A few years ago, Lucinda, a partner in a law firm, came in to have her eyes done. Pleased with the results, she returned for a brow-lift. At about the same time, I was seeing another lawyer, Helen, who had quite a bit of work done: first her brow, eyes, and face, and then a tummy tuck.

About a year after these two women had done their procedures, I was walking down the hall when I heard Lucinda say, "Oh, my God, Helen, what are you doing here? I just left you at the office." It turned out that Lucinda and Helen were close friends who ate lunch together as often as they could. Lucinda had told Helen all about her surgery, but Helen had never wanted to tell Lucinda. Lorraine told me later that Helen was nearly apoplectic with worry by the time Lorraine hustled her into the privacy of a consult room.

"Don't say anything to Lucinda," Helen begged her. "We have to think of why I'm here. She's going to be so mad at me for not telling her."

They decided that the best cover was to pretend that Helen was there because she was considering getting Botox injections. Lucinda believed her. And Helen heaved a huge sigh of relief that her secret was safe.

My office staff always tries to keep people who know one another from arriving at the same time, but that's sometimes impossible—we don't always know which patients know one another. And many do, of course, because most of my practice is based on word-of-mouth referrals. But just because someone passes along the name of a plastic surgeon to her best friend doesn't mean the best friend will confess to having ever made an appointment . . . much less scheduling a procedure.

Here are three of my typical patients who decided to take the plunge.

Leslie: It's Now or Never

Leslie, now fifty-five, had come to me a year earlier to talk about what a face-lift could do for her. After a pleasant conversation, she didn't book the surgery, and I figured I would never see her again. Yet now, here she was, still wrestling with the same questions.

"I have to tell you," she said, "it's which way the wind's blowing. But I've made a decision. If I'm going to do it, I'm doing it this year, because I'm sick of looking like an old hag!"

I laughed. "You certainly don't look like an old hag, and your hesitation is perfectly normal and perfectly valid. I can say, however, that the likelihood of a major problem happening is very, very remote," I said, hoping to allay her fears. "I've been doing this for sixteen years and I haven't had a major bad thing happen. A lot of the reason why is patient selection. I don't do a face-lift on a woman who's seventy-five years old and put her under for up to six hours."

"I'm not worried about dying," Leslie said with a little shrug. "I'm worried about how I'll look when it's over. I don't want to have a face that looks forty-five and a body that looks sixty-five. And my hands have always looked old to me too. Can you do a hand-lift at the same time?"

"I wish I could."

"Oh, well." She sighed deeply. "I don't care that they look like old hands," she went on, "but I don't want it to be like, someone sees your face and then your hands and says, 'Oh, my God, *of course* she had a face-lift.'"

"A light peel or a bleaching cream could make your hands a little better, but unfortunately there's not much else we can do for them now," I said. "Only you can decide whether your overall look will be wrong."

"What would be the minimum, and what would be the maximum?"

"I see a couple of things," I told her. In her jaw, there was a little bit of jowling. "Open your eyes and look at me." I examined her carefully. "Your lower eyelids are fine, although they could use a little resurfacing with laser to eliminate the fine lines. With your upper eyelids, it's a combination of the position of the brow and a little extra skin. The maximum, or ideal situation, for that is an endoscopic brow-lift. At the same time I'd trim a little skin from the upper eyelids. That's the maximum for the upper third of your face.

"On the lower two-thirds, you have a couple of platysmal bands in the neck, which are the platysmal muscle. To fix them requires a face-lift. Even when you're relaxed, those two bands are quite visible, which is relatively unusual in someone your age. Through a small incision I would tighten the muscle, then redrape the skin and cut the excess. That's the maximum. That would include, of course, lifting the malar fat pads in your cheeks to make your face look younger."

I looked to see if she wanted me to go on.

"And what's the minimum?" Leslie asked.

"On your lower lids, if those lines bother you, laser resurfacing is the only way to go. On your uppers, I think trimming the skin is reasonable. My job is obviously to tell you what I'm seeing. Otherwise I'm not doing my job."

"If you said I could do it right now, I would sign up," she said.

"You have good bone structure, so you should have terrific results. In someone who has a lot of fat, it's difficult to get a contoured neck. But you don't have that problem."

"What will a face-lift do to my lips?"

"It will slightly elevate the corners. The pull should be no more than forty-five degrees along the angle of the jaw."

She sighed again. "What's really nagging me is what happened to my friend Louise. She had a brow-lift and her eyes done, and now she can't completely close her eyes. She has to put gunk in her eyes every night. She was beautiful, and now she looks terrible."

"Too much skin was obviously taken out of the upper eyelid," I explained. "That hasn't happened to me in sixteen years of practice."

"I came to you because I trust you a hundred percent," Leslie said, rubbing her hands along her neck. "It's just that I can't stop obsessing about Louise's eyes. If you do all these procedures simultaneously, does it open up the potential for error?"

"Yes, and no. Theoretically it does, but at this point in my life, I have the judgment not to overdo it."

And at a certain point, taking the plunge is no longer about rationality or logic. You just have to give in and say yes. I trust this doctor. I'm going to do it.

Which is exactly what Leslie said.

And then she told me her only regret was that she hadn't done it ten years before.

Cindy: A Forehead of Wrinkles

Cindy had her breasts enlarged a decade ago and has been coming to me for Botox injections in her forehead for the last three years. She is forty-four, very fit, a weight lifter with biceps bulkier than Madonna's, a wonderfully toned body, and the energy (not to mention flirtatiousness) that makes her agelessly appealing. But her forehead wrinkles were annoying her, and the cost of the shots was adding up. Three years of Botox is more expensive than having a brow surgically corrected, a procedure that will probably last for eight or nine years. I knew she wanted a brow-lift but was hesitating partly because of the cost.

I asked her if she would like to be the subject of a presentation I was scheduled to give to a conference of plastic surgeons called "The Cutting Edge IV," sponsored by Manhattan Eye, Ear and Throat Hospital. No one would know her name, and her face would never be shown directly. Only her forehead. My surgical fee would be waived, and she'd have to pay only for the hospital room and the anesthesia. That basically cut the price in half.

Cindy nearly fell off her chair in excitement. It was the exact incentive she needed.

It was videotaped at Manhattan Eye and Ear, and everything went perfectly. I did an endoscopic brow-lift and an upper blepheroplasty, taking fat out of the upper eyelids. When Cindy woke up after the surgery, she was thrilled. Her forehead was smooth.

Four days later, she came to my office for the mandatory checkup, and now she wasn't so thrilled. In fact, she was nearly hysterical. Her best friend, Shelley, who'd picked her up after surgery and had been taking care of her, sat next to her, stroking her hand. Cindy looked like a battered woman. Her eyes were intensely black and blue, and her entire face was grotesquely swollen. Even though I warn patients of potential surgical aftereffects, they almost always assume that nothing will happen to them.

Until it happens.

"Is this *really* normal?" she asked frantically, very unlike her usual in-control and pragmatic self. "Yesterday it was so cool. I had no swelling."

"I know. But this is normal. It's not a big deal."

On the intercom I called the nurse and asked her to bring in an ice pack, so Cindy could start icing even before she left the office.

"You swear this is normal?"

"How long have you known me? Ten years? Trust me, if I thought something was wrong, I would most certainly tell you. Your swelling is a little worse than the average, but you're well within the norm. Just ice it. Within a day you'll see a big difference."

The ice pack arrived, and I told her to put it against her face. She looked at the ice pack and started laughing, more like her old self. "This has your name on it," she said. "You're nuts. I wouldn't think you'd exactly want me to be your surgery poster child right now." She pressed the ice close to her forehead. "I never get bruised, you know. This is totally freaking me out. Look. Even my scars from when you did my breasts healed without a hitch." She started to lift up her shirt.

"When women start showing me their bodies, I get totally discombobulated," I said, laughing. "But I believe you."

I had a nurse in the room, so I didn't have to worry about anything untoward happening. And I knew Cindy wasn't that kind of patient, anyway.

"Once, a woman came to me for collagen injections for some deep lines on her face that were bothering her," I told Cindy and Shelley. "I went into the examining room, and did a double take because she'd already taken her top off. She was just sitting there without a care in the world. 'What do you think of my breasts?' she asked.

" 'I'll get your collagen,' I muttered and I ran out. When I went back, I had the nurse with me.

"So, tell me," I said. "What did you do yesterday?"

"We watched television, and I had a nice long bath," she replied.

"Was it a warm bath?" I asked. She nodded. *Eureka!*

"That was definitely not a good idea," I said. "Hot baths cause vasodilation, which increases swelling. It's not unusual to get more swollen the second day, so as I said, this is normal, but no more baths. You'll make it worse. You can wash your hair if you're desperate, but only baby shampoo. No conditioner. No hair products. *Nothing* near your brow. Be careful, because you have staples in your scalp, and a lot of gunk." She'd had two incisions about two inches back from the start of her hairline, closed up with staples instead of stitches, that are taken out after a week.

Patients hate it when I tell them to leave their hair alone after surgery. No products, no mousse, no spray, and most definitely no color for at least three to four weeks.

And no cheating.

"You'll look both better and worse as the week wears on," I explained. "Thanks to gravity, all of the fluid goes down. So your eyes will start to look better, but by the next time I see you in a few days, you'll have a little bit of a jowl. That's also perfectly normal and will soon go away."

When I saw Cindy at her next appointment, she looked great.

"Your incisions are healing incredibly well. It must be your nice clean lifestyle," I teased.

"Oh, yeah?" she retorted. "Did I ever tell you about the time I had sex on the desk of my boyfriend's office? Of course, now he's not my boyfriend. He's my husband."

I laughed. "That reminds me of the tale of the plastic surgeon who was caught having sex on his desk at work with someone who wasn't his wife . . . by his wife. You never know. One of my patients earlier today was as seemingly proper as they come," I went on. "Her first and only question was how quickly she could have sex after her tummy tuck. She was hoping I would say three days."

Cindy laughed too. "So tell me, was my swelling *really* normal?"

"There's a curve," I replied. "You were a little bit past the median, so you looked more beaten up than average. If you're not used to any bruising or swelling, it can be scary, but it truly does take two full weeks to recover to the point where no one will notice."

She sighed deeply in relief. "I never should have taken that bath," she admitted.

"But that's no reason to make yourself a prisoner," I went on. "With a little makeup, you can go anywhere."

"That day I came in here with my eyes such a mess, Shelley was crying more than me because I was so black and blue," she said. "You know how we are about our looks."

"You're lucky to have such a great friend."

"I know. And you're lucky that Shelley's going to make an appointment to come see you about getting liposuction on her thighs," she said with another laugh.

A few days later, I knew Cindy must really have been happy with her looks, because she brought me a piece of artwork she had done, a surrealist piece with the head from a Leonardo portrait superimposed on an etching of a forest. The note read, "Love, Cindy." To me, that's the most meaningful present of all, something that shows a patient appreciates my sense of artistry in what I did with her.

Susan: The Drooping Lid

At first, Susan, a photographer, thought she had a neurological problem with her eyes. She'd been seeing shadows when she worked. Sometimes she'd get the feeling that somebody was coming up behind her, often from the right.

Susan, fifty-three, was charmingly outspoken, pretty, although slightly worn out looking, as if she'd spent far too many years basking and partying in the sun.

"I kept thinking this is weird," she said. "So, okay, I used to be a sun goddess. Was I having a stroke? But then I realized my lids were drooping so far down that they were starting to cover my lashes. That's why I'm here."

"Let me take a look," I said. "Relax your forehead." I immediately saw that although she did have excess skin on her lids, her brow had also descended significantly. She was continually lifting her brows and wrinkling her forehead in an attempt to open up her field of vision.

"To correct your upper eyelid, I'd have to do a couple of things. Your brow has to be repositioned, lifted only three millimeters or so. It isn't a lot, but it makes a difference. The second thing is to put an incision in the natural crease of the lid and remove the fat and excess skin. After a few months, you won't even see the incision in your lid. The brow-lift is a more significant surgery, but the scars will be hidden under your hair. And, as you know, your lower lids are also very full. Do they bother you?"

"Well, I'd like to have my whole face done, but we don't have that much money," she said. "Does it look funny when you do only the top and not the bottom?"

I nodded. "It does a bit. I understand that the upper half of your face has the real problem, but you do have some fullness on the bottom that can easily be rectified."

"What I'd like," she said, "is a little gusset with a collar so you could just pull it all up. This gravity stuff is hard to take. It sucks."

I smiled. "Yes, gravity does suck. I couldn't have said it better myself."

After our consultation, she scheduled surgery on her forehead and upper lids, because for her, doing nothing wasn't an option. She had to take the plunge to make the shadows clouding her vision go away. After her endoscopic brow-lift, she'll look as if someone has slightly lifted her forehead and thinned out her eyelids. Not radically different, but better. Rested, more alert. She'll also look a lot happier, because a descending brow tends to make people look fierce.

Ten

WHAT I DIDN'T LEARN DURING MY TRAINING IS ENOUGH TO FILL A BOOK

Sex and the Surgeon

I've never dated patients. The temptations could have been overwhelming—if I'd been looking for that sort of *je ne sais quoi* en route to a face-lift.

The reasons they weren't overwhelming for me is that Lorraine has been part of my life for fifteen years, and we've been happily married for eight years. But even when I was single, I always heard plenty of scary stories.

And the person who usually got screwed wasn't the patient.

One surgeon started dating a woman who'd come to him for a rhinoplasty. Things were moving along nicely, but then he decided she wasn't the one. He broke up with her, and she was not happy about it. She started complaining about her nose. She started threatening a lawsuit. She kept complaining, making his life miserable. She wouldn't have been able to do that if he'd maintained a purely professional relationship. He would have been able to say, "Sue me, or don't sue me. I know my work is impeccable." Chances are she would have dropped it.

But once you expose yourself to the possibility of a compromised position and questionable ethics—after all, it can be argued that any doctor dating a patient is taking advantage of a very real vulnerability—you may well have to pay the price.

Even doctors who aren't interested in dating patients should certainly maintain the utmost professional demeanor to create safeguards against potential misunderstandings. A surgeon I knew on the West Coast was incredibly nice by nature. He worked on the eyes of a female patient, who not so subtly dropped a few hints during her follow-up visits that she'd like to see him socially. He graciously declined, telling her that he was married.

But she wouldn't take no for an answer. She found out where he lived and started sending letters to his house and calling him in the middle of the night. He had to go to the police and eventually obtained a restraining order against her.

She retaliated by suing him for sexual harassment, claiming that he fondled her breasts while he was marking up her face for her eye surgery. There'd been no one else in the room at the time, so it was a she-said-he-said kind of situation. It actually ended up in court, and although he was exonerated in the end because she had no proof to back up her accusation, it shattered his nerves and his confidence, ruining both his career and his love of treating patients. Thoroughly disillusioned, he quit being a surgeon. All because of a vindictive patient who felt rejected.

Every doctor worries about such a worst-case scenario with a deranged patient, which is why I always have a female assistant in the room with me when I meet with female patients. I don't want to take the chance of something that devastating happening to me. With a witness to back me up, it can't. That may sound paranoid, but I don't think any male doctor in any specialty should be in a room with a door closed and a female patient in some state of undress.

Not all patient-doctor encounters have unseemly endings. Plenty of single (or not so single) plastic surgeons date their patients. They consider themselves lucky to have an endless stream of attractive women who may send out obvious signals during consultations.

And it must be said that many female patients do throw themselves at their doctors. They aren't interested in lawsuits. They're interested in fun. Plus they get a crush on the one who made them look beautiful. They glorify us and praise us, and I'd be lying if I said it wasn't a nice stroke for the ego. It can be hard to resist.

But I have always resisted, because I think it's unethical to date any patient. As I said, patients are always in an inherently vulnerable position. They need to trust their doctor. Will the patient feel she has to have sex in order to get a good surgical result or a good follow-up? Is she angling for free work in the future?

Of course, I don't see a problem with an unattached doctor and patient dating once the professional relationship has ended.

Just be sure it really *has* ended.

How to Talk to Patients

Human interaction is a huge part of being a doctor that never gets discussed during medical school or residency. Having a successful bedside (or officeside) manner is not taught. And it should be. Too many doctors I know are brusque, or inconsiderate of patients' emotional needs and worries, or just plain rude. It took me a while to figure out how best to approach my patients.

Paramount is treating every patient with respect.

I talk differently with every patient, depending on the cues they throw out. Over the years, I've honed my instincts down to a science, and I've learned how to alter my conversation and level of seriousness depending on the personality of my patient. I throw out a conversational line and see where it goes. I don't joke with those who are serious by inclination. I don't belittle or discount any fears or nervousness anyone has.

And if women want to flirt, I flirt. Just a little, to keep the banter lively and help them relax.

Men don't usually want to talk about personal things the way women do. We often talk about cars and speed, which is fine with me, because I love my Porsche and my Harley Heritage Softtail motorcycle. I often tell them about the time I rode my chopper to Boston for a plastic surgery conference. I was going to give a presentation, and my slides were in the saddlebag. I rode up to the Four Seasons in Copley Square, and the door-man looked at me like, What the hell are *you* doing in a fancy hotel. He asked if I was a guest, and I told him I was. Then he told me I couldn't park my motorcycle there. I said, "Well, then would you mind parking it for me?"

The look on his face was priceless.

How to Schedule Patients

I used to treat the ex-wife of a famous rock and roller. Even though they'd been divorced for a number of years, she was furious that his career had soared after they broke up. She'd stand in the office and yell, "That fucking guy couldn't even get it up when we were married, let alone have an affair." And so on and so forth.

Her appointment was always scheduled to be either the first or the last of the day so she wouldn't bother the other patients with her tirades.

Anyone who veers from the usual patient lineup—the extremely ner-vous, the extremely talkative, the extremely obnoxious—usually gets scheduled for the first or last appointment. It's not fair to everyone else to have what should be a pleasant and comfortable wait marred by some-one else's problems.

I also learned it's never a good idea to have exotic dancers sharing the waiting room with the Park Avenue ladies who lunch.

Many years ago, one of my favorite patients was an exotic dancer named Sheila. "Honey," she said, "fuck that exotic dancer shit. I'm a stripper and proud of it!" To say she was flamboyant is an understatement—she made sure she owned every room she entered in a sexual way, always wearing very short skirts and very high heels, with her breasts hanging out of whatever bit of fabric she chose to wear that day. So when she'd come in with some of the girls she danced with, we'd close the office to the rest of the patients. Sheila's girlfriends and fellow strippers would sprawl all over the sofas, the breasts I'd enhanced falling out of their tops, their voices raspy from the cigarettes they'd try to sneak when the staff wasn't looking. They'd all crowd into an examining room and take their clothes off at the same time. For some reason, all my friends wanted to assist me at those sessions.

Sheila liked to tease me that she'd written my name on the wall in one of the topless clubs where they danced.

I'd much rather treat a stripper who's happy with my work than a suburbanite who isn't.

How to Deal with Angry Patients

Rosie had been taking the Metro North train in to the city for collagen injections for eight years. When I was just establishing my practice I had no trouble with her. The office was not overcrowded, so she never had to wait. But over time, that has changed.

I can't always keep exactly to the appointment schedule. Some sessions take longer than expected, and there is no way to anticipate that. If people are frustrated by the wait and leave, we call them and apologize, and offer another appointment. If they stay—and most do—I make it clear when I walk into the examining room that I'm sorry. I tell them I'm trying to see patients as quickly as possible, but sometimes it takes longer than anticipated. If I'm late from surgery, I tell them that I know they wouldn't want me to hurry through *their* surgeries. Nearly all my patients understand that this is just the way things are, and I never *want* to keep anyone waiting.

Rosie didn't care about that. She was so furious about having to wait that she made a big scene in the waiting room. Lorraine whisked her into a consulting room so she wouldn't disturb all the other waiting patients, and we let it go at that. But the next time she came, she stood at the desk complaining loudly about her bill, trying to finagle down the cost. It was embarrassing with all of the other patients listening.

We sent her a letter after that telling her that we appreciated patients who would not disrupt the office decorum, and that she knew our prices were fixed and not negotiable. She was fine after that.

HOW TO TELL WHEN A PATIENT IS LYING

- She tells me she has never had a face-lift and I see unfortunate, big scars around her ears.
- He tells me he doesn't smoke, but I can smell it on his clothes the minute he walks into the examining room.
- She tells me she is in perfect health, but then the presurgery physical shows she can't walk up two flights of stairs without becoming seriously winded.
- He says he has never had a serious health problem, and then the physical reveals that he is on blood pressure medication.
- She said at least three times during all the presurgical consultations that she doesn't take any medication, but just before the anesthesiologist starts the drugs needed for surgery she whispers that she occasionally takes an antidepressant.
- I ask her how old she is, and she answers by asking, "How old do you think I am?" (This falls into the lying-by-evasion category.)
- He says he has never used cocaine, but I'm looking at a huge hole in the septum of his nose that couldn't have been caused by anything else.
- She's dripping in diamonds and complains loudly in the waiting room that she can't afford the cost of a Botox injection.
- He apologizes for always being late by explaining that his driver got a speeding ticket.
- She says she's never been to another plastic surgeon after I've seen her face being worked on in the hospital, on the table in the operating room of one of my colleagues.

Personal Style: Your Office and Your Suit as a Sales Tool

There's a certain pressure to being a member of the Park Avenue Posse that is completely unrelated to the medical pressure.

It's the pressure to find the right interior decorator.

We all attract different types of patients with our offices and with our personalities. My residents tell me they can figure out which plastic surgeon is working on which patient at the hospital that day—before they even look at the chart—just by the patient's personality. Stuffed shirts go to Dr. X. Rhinoplasty junkies go to Dr. Y. Demanding rich women go to Dr. Z. I get a lot of self-made people, often in the arts and music, who tend to be on the young side. I think my office has something to do with it.

Your office is as much your sales tool as your Savile Row suit. Looks do matter. For me, this isn't easy. My own inclination is to dress down. I love my comfortable scrubs and could happily see patients in them all day. That's never gone down well with Lorraine, and I have to admit she has a point. This is a service business. My patients are paying a lot of money for Park Avenue service, and they are going to get it. I have to look Park Avenue and act Park Avenue too. Lorraine knows that every prospective patient will be judging me by the appearance of my office, and, whether he or she knows it or not, by my face, by my shoes, and by the cut of my suit. Every visual cue gives off subtle messages about my aesthetic judgment—and also shows how different I am from other plastic surgeons.

My wife has a fit when I try to sneak out of the house on weekends to buy the newspapers if I'm wearing a pair of bicycle shorts and my favorite crummy Onion Heads T-shirt. If a patient walked by and saw me in that getup, I might be humiliated.

I have to concede that she has a point.

My wife also says I shouldn't be loud and brawling in restaurants on the Upper East Side with my friends, because patients might see me there too. Not that I'm loud or a brawler, but again, she's right. There are always photographers lurking around in New York, looking for gossip. Doctors who've acted out their personal dramas and problems in public have seen their faces splashed and reputations impugned in the papers, sometimes for weeks on end. That's not going to happen to me.

And when it comes to our waiting rooms, most of the Park Avenue Posse have lushly furnished, fairly traditional offices that speak quietly yet luxuriously of serious money. Plastic surgeons, not surprisingly, are visually oriented. We're much more likely than other doctors to get involved in the design of decorative items for our offices, and in the details, because it matters tremendously to us. We're competing among ourselves with our offices, too, which doctors who aren't in a visual field need not do. People shop for plastic surgeons; they don't shop in the same way for other kinds of doctors. They're mostly well off, and if they have to pay a few consulting fees to find someone they like, it's usually not the end of the world to them. And since they shop around, they're choosing partly on how comfortable they feel in an office.

Waiting rooms usually have a plush sofa, a few upholstered chairs, simple yet stylish objets d'art, and lavishly bound presentation books of the doctor's press clippings and before-and-after photographs of his or her handiwork. We want people to feel comfortable. Some offices serve coffee; others have phones. There should be a pleasant receptionist with a well-modulated voice asking whether she can help. Behind her are the examining rooms and, in many cases, the surgical suites.

I was lucky to have found a terrific architect, Karen Jacobson, to take charge of my office. She's often worked with plastic surgeons and understood that I wanted my place to be different, to reflect my taste, my interest in modern art, my appreciation for clean lines. I didn't want that overstuffed, plush Ralph Lauren look, not that there is anything wrong with that. I'd been out one night in the Tribeca Grand Hotel for drinks and suddenly realized that I wanted my office to look like that—a sleek, streamlined, modern hotel.

Karen told me that most of the Park Avenue Posse want their offices to reflect their confidence and to give the image that they have arrived. Their offices often resemble their Park Avenue apartments: traditional, classy and, to my way of thinking, a bit boring. Certainly not sleek and sophisticated.

When Karen was finished, my office was the ultimate in cool, the epitome of a minimalist space using metal, wood, and glass. She also told me that after renovations of plastic surgeons' offices, their business has gone way up.

That's certainly what happened to me.

Here's a tip: In their private offices, most surgeons have photographs of their families. Their wives have inevitably been operated on. I'm not making fun of anyone here. My wife has had surgery.

You can tell a lot about a surgeon by looking at his wife. If she is over-pulled or overdone, chances are high that you will be too. I know a surgeon whose wife is a victim of excess operations. Her face has no expression, her lips are overdone, and her breasts are out to there. To me, she's a caricature of what beauty should be. But in a way, she's a walking advertisement for her husband, and he obviously wants to project that image. There will always be some surgeons who believe that more is better.

Let them believe it. It's not for me.

Watch Out for Your Ego

Ego Management 101. That's the one class in medical school everyone should attend . . . but never did and never will.

Doctors do understand that their egos can be a problem. That said, egos can still blow up into monstrous proportions. There are far too many plastic surgeons who think they're God. Their grateful patients worship them. Women fall in love with them. Their workers bow down to them. I've had patients who've come into my office and said, "You've changed my life. You're my hero. You're my god. Tell me what I can do for you." They send me gifts. They send me letters.

I think ego management is very different for other specialists. When you have your gallbladder out, sure you're grateful. You're happy you didn't die. You say, thank heaven that's over. And that's it.

Plastic surgery is not like that. People come out transformed. Plus I often see patients for years, and they're grateful that I'm keeping them looking the way they want to look. That's something they think about every time they look in a mirror.

You have to step back and have a reality check. It would be a problem if I started believing in my own "godlike" qualities. There are doctors who do, and their heads become so big they can hardly carry them. They start treating their families and their staffs terribly. Patients pick up on that, and I think they begin to resent it when they sense that their doctor's ego is out of control.

My motto is: Swollen heads come after face-lifts.

Not after seeing patients.

How to Have a Good Eye

Surgeons don't learn to be visual in medical school. They don't learn to have an eye. It must be instinct. All of us can pick up the same set of technical skills during our training, but without an appropriate sense of what is beautiful, and the eye to know when to stop, the tools can do more harm than good.

Along with an innate sense of aesthetics, it helps to have a unique way of looking at the world, in every dimension, because so much of plastic surgery is sculptural in nature. I was lucky that my parents always stressed the importance of art and culture, and museum going has long been an important part of my life.

Either you have it or you don't. When I scrub with a new resident, I know within ten minutes whether he or she will be a good surgeon or a mediocre one. It's not the technical skills I notice. Those can be taught and always improved upon. Teaching aesthetic judgment is very difficult, if not impossible. There are surgeons who go way overboard in their surgery, who really make people look worse, and they're not necessarily badly educated. Some of them write and lecture. They know their stuff. But if their sense of aesthetics is off, then the surgery will not be a true success.

What differentiates the top surgeons from the average surgeons is the instinctive knack for that visual harmony.

Of course, having a killer technique doesn't mean you'll have a killer practice. As you've already figured out.

The Learning Curve Never Ends, and You're a Fool if You Think It Does

I had the best training that was available for all the years I was in medical school and doing my advanced studies with the best teachers in the world.

Most of it is now completely outdated.

We're not talking about decades ago. I've been in practice for only sixteen years. In the scope of a career, that's not long. But most of the procedures I do today were not taught to me in medical school, or even during my residency. I had to learn how to do them by studying, watching more experienced surgeons, or just figuring it out myself. There are still doctors who don't do certain procedures, because they don't know how to do them.

Being a plastic surgeon must be an ongoing learning process. You can learn all the basic techniques during your training, but you have to learn to apply them in new ways. You have to be continually willing to learn, relearn, and improve your moves during surgery.

Be sure to ask your surgeon how often he refreshes his knowledge. It's a valid question, and you should get a straight answer.

If you don't, find a doctor less willing to rest on his laurels and more willing to open his mind.

Running a Business

I had no concept of how to run a business when I started my own. I didn't know how to establish a practice; I didn't know how to hire and fire staff. I had no idea about insurance issues, or even how to submit a bill to an insurance company. Now there are some courses like that in medical school, but there weren't when I was there, so I had no idea. Absolutely none.

I had to learn from my mistakes. One of my most important lessons was always to get the money first. Before I operate on someone, I require cash, a check, or a credit card. No excuses.

I got burned once when I first started out—by a former nun, of all people. She came in for eyelid surgery. In the course of conversation, it came out that she'd been in a convent. She seemed nice enough. She was supposed to pay two weeks in advance, but no check showed up. When you first start your own practice, *any* case is a great case, so I didn't want to lose it. When she apologized and said she'd bring the check to the surgery, I said fine, as long as it was a certified check. When she showed up with a personal check, I was leery, but I was still too green to cancel her operation. Which is what I should have done. But I figured, would a former nun stiff me?

Two days after the procedure, I saw her in my office to take out the external sutures.

"I'm not happy," she said as she sat down.

"I'm sorry to hear that," I said. "But it's too soon really to be unhappy. You have no idea how good you're going to look when the swelling goes down."

I saw her again two days later to take out the last of the stitches. Later that afternoon, I found out that her check had bounced. In those days, $3,500 was a lot of money for me. It more than paid the rent in my office. That was the very last time I ever took a personal check, unless of course it is given to me two weeks before and has time to clear.

So I got stiffed by a former nun, and she had the nerve to complain.

Now, if there's no payment, I say good-bye.

Friends as Patients, Patients as Friends

Unlike many in the Park Avenue Posse, I don't socialize with patients. I never talk about surgery when I'm out. It can be risky. I almost got slapped once by a woman I'd just met when I answered her question about what work she might need done.

I've never made that mistake again. I've become friends with only a few patients. It's something I don't encourage.

Although I like to joke around with many of my patients I've seen over the years, and sometimes talk about personal things, I still think it's prudent to keep a certain distance from patients when I'm outside of the office. It's blurring the ethical line.

Friends as patients are an entirely different matter. I operate on a lot of my friends, and it can be a problem. There comes a time when there are so many friends and so many who want something. Lorraine and I are starting to realize that some of the people who called themselves our friends also want free surgery or injections. It's never really discussed aloud. But when our friends come in, they know we're not going to make them pay. They say, "Oh, just charge me." Or "Make sure you send me a bill." But they never pull out a checkbook and say, "How much do I owe you?" It's getting more complicated, because it takes up time, time that I could be using to make a living.

Let's face it, I can afford to do free procedures. By the same token, my friends can usually afford to pay retail. Still, they shouldn't get something for nothing. I'm thinking of saying, "Look, this is a five-thousand-dollar procedure, and of course I'm not charging you. Instead, I'd like a check for twenty-five hundred made out to a charity—maybe an organization of plastic surgeons that does reconstructive work for children in the third world."

My friends will get surgery and will have done a good deed, and a child in Guatemala will no longer have a cleft palate.

But I think I might have to ask them to hand Lorraine the check before surgery. Otherwise those kids might not get their transformations.

Eleven

HEAD LINES: BROWS, EYES, NOSES, AND FACE-LIFTS

THAT VOICE WAS UNMISTAKABLE. I KNEW IT WAS KATHARINE HEPBURN before she said her name. She'd gotten my number from Sherrell Aston's office. He was her doctor but was out of town. Back then, in 1989, I often got his referrals. Miss Hepburn needed an immediate appointment because a friend had cut a leg on a fence on the Hepburn estate in eastern Connecticut. I told her to come in right away. She sat on the sofa for two hours, patiently waiting while I fixed the gash on her friend's leg.

A year later, Dr. Aston called and said that Miss Hepburn had a basal cell carcinoma, a fairly common type of skin cancer, on her face, and it needed to be removed. Another surgeon, Dr. Mike Albom, would remove the cancer, and he thought I should do the reconstruction. At that point, I had been out on my own for about five years and was still considered a newcomer, so I was thrilled with his confidence in me as well as the opportunity to work on such a famous face.

The operation was performed at Manhattan Eye and Ear, in Operating Room 2. Dr. Aston was working on one of his patients in Room One, and Dr. Michael Hogan, one of the senior surgeons, was operating on someone else in Room Three.

I watched eagerly as Dr. Albom began work on Miss Hepburn's face. I could see that her cancer was right between the nose and the mouth, in the nasolabial fold. He began cutting, and after taking out a bit, sent it to the lab for analysis. He resected—which means cut away tissue—again and found that it was still positive for cancer. He resected again. Still cancer. He had made the third pass, and she was still not free of the cancer. He resected for the fourth time.

By then he had taken out a significant portion of the cheek and was encroaching on the eyelids. I was starting to worry. I knew that she was scheduled soon to shoot a television special. Dr. Aston kept popping in and out, not saying anything, just shaking his head. Here was one of the most recognizable faces in the world, and Dr. Albom had to keep going until all the cancer was gone. By now, half her nose and cheek had been affected.

Dr. Hogan came in and looked at her. He blanched. "Paul, you got a problem," he said. And walked out.

Dr. Aston came in again and looked at her. "What are you going to do?" he asked. And he walked out too.

It was a difficult situation. Here I was, trying to make a name for myself in a competitive market, faced with a gaping wound on Katharine Hepburn's beloved face. Dr. Aston didn't do that kind of reconstructive work. And nobody else had done hundreds of cases like this one either, because the placement and depth of her cancer were uncommon. This kind of work is fascinating for someone like me, of course, but it's also extremely complicated and difficult. I'd have to make an incision similar to what's done for a face-lift and then rotate the whole face. It would take at least several hours and require a complicated thought process, because there is no standard way of doing it. You have to adjust as you go. If you don't do it exactly right you can lose the whole flap of rotated skin, and it will die. That would be a nightmare, necessitating skin grafts and possibly leading to substantial scarring.

Thankfully, I did a very good job. Miss Hepburn ended up looking great. The scars healed perfectly.

My reward was that after the surgery, I got to make house calls at Miss Hepburn's town house on Forty-ninth Street in Manhattan and during the recuperation period make sure that she was healing correctly. Her secretary always made me lunch, and then Miss Hepburn and I would sit and talk—about everything. Her father had been a neurosurgeon, and she would tell me she understood that what I did was very difficult and time-consuming. She really was partial to physicians. During our talks, I never pried into her life. We never talked about Spencer Tracy, or about the movies, as I didn't think those topics were appropriate. And she never referred to being a movie star, or acted like a movie star. For someone who was such a legend, Katharine Hepburn was the sweetest, most wonderful person, without a pretentious bone in her body.

I operated on her several times after that for skin cancer. She healed well every time. For her, having cancer was a nuisance. For me, it was always a thrill hearing that famous voice.

Of course, if she were still alive, I wouldn't be telling this story and using her name.

Few facial cases have ever come as close to that drama with Miss Hepburn, but as much close attention and concentration must be paid during every procedure. Plastic surgeons who have a cavalier attitude toward any work done on the face should have their heads examined!

If mistakes are made on the body, at least you have the option of covering it up. If mistakes are made on the face, the entire world can see your misfortune. Patients are beyond distraught. They're devastated.

If you've chosen your surgeon carefully, you shouldn't have to worry, though. Facial procedures are increasingly common and popular, so let's talk about brow-lifts, eye procedures, nose jobs, and face-lifts. In recent years, refinements to technique have greatly improved surgery, reducing the potential for visible scarring as well as the recuperation time. This is especially true for brow-lifts.

A Bunch of Deadheads: The Endoscopic Brow-Lift

Warning: Graphic material ahead. Skip to the next section if you're squeamish.

When I was training to be a plastic surgeon, brow-lifts weren't subtle.

The standard procedure was to make an incision from ear to ear and then lift the skin up from the bone, which we call undermining, along the entire forehead.

I was never crazy about that procedure, which hadn't really been improved upon since it had been introduced in the 1930s, so I started trying to figure out a better way to do the brow-lift. In the early 1990s, there was growing interest in endoscopic surgery on all parts of the body. An endoscope is a device containing a small camera, which can project images on a computer screen. By moving the scope around inside the body, surgeons can see a large area, and by working through a small incision with that extensive view, they can do operations that would once have required large incisions. In 1992, I heard about someone in California who was working on techniques for using the endoscope in face-lifts. I remember telling Sherrell Aston that it sounded so out there, I thought we should investigate if it was feasible or not.

He agreed. After all, the credo of the plastic surgeon is to minimize scarring, and the work we were doing on foreheads led to large scars from ear to ear. In addition, because the scars were closed up under tension, patients often got numbness or funny feelings near their scalps, as well as occasional hair loss.

I wanted to learn more about the relationship between the nerves and the musculature in the forehead. Oddly, very little research had been done on that. At the time, I was a young attending surgeon at Manhattan Eye and Ear, four years into my practice. I examined the underlying structure of the foreheads carefully in the next twenty brow-lifts that I did, as well as the ones Aston did. When the skin flap was down during surgery, I would measure everything so I could study the relative placements of nerve and muscle. I presented a paper on "The Course and Relation of Sensory Nerves of the Forehead" to the 1993 annual meeting of the American Society for Aesthetic Plastic Surgery, which brought me an award for the best scientific exhibit that year at the society's meeting. In November 1993, I heard that someone in Baltimore was trying to do endoscopic brow-lifts. By then, I was eager to see if it was possible. But we couldn't start experimenting on patients. We needed a dissection.

Dissections are done on cadavers. If you're a doctor, you can buy a torso, or a head, or whatever you need. Actually, you don't *buy* them. You pay to use them.

The going rate for a cadaver head in 1993 was $400.

In medical school, you work on bodies that have been preserved with formaldehyde. But the cadaver heads we got were better. They'd been fresh frozen. Working on them feels very different, much more lifelike.

I told you this section isn't for the squeamish!

The heads were delivered to us at the hospital by one of the companies that supply cadaver parts. I'll never forget the name of the woman who brought them: Beth. Beth and her boyfriend would drive around in a truck with these dead heads in the back. We had to sign an agreement that we would not dissect the whole face, just the forehead so that other doctors could use the heads later for different dissections.

Dr. Aston and I took the heads into the basement of the hospital one night and went to work in an anatomy lab, which was more often used for drilling into the ear by residents learning about bone structure. I felt like Frankenstein, hunched over a severed head in a basement late at night.

And then we really got going. Using a scalpel, we made two small slits in the hair, then put in the endoscope and began the procedure. After doing a few dissections, I flew out to La Jolla at the end of 1993 for the first course given on this technique by Dr. Nicanor Isse. He and his colleagues were also investigating how best to use the scope, and I learned a lot from their progress. When I got back to New York, we gave our own course. Once we started using the procedure on live patients, I quickly found how valuable it could be. It was a huge advance over the old technique, because it eliminated both scarring and hair loss.

Using the endoscope to see where I was going, I could separate the skin of the forehead from the underlying muscle and fascia, going right down to the orbital rim (the eye socket). To make everything mobile, I would cut the galea, the fibrous tissue that lies just above the periosteum, which is the layer that covers the bone. Thanks to what I'd learned in my previous research, I was easily able to identify the nerves, which look like a white, yellowish strand. It was important to locate them early on, so I could avoid hitting them and causing permanent damage. I could identify the muscle and begin removing it.

That's basically how the brow-lift works. Once the muscles that depress the brow are eliminated or weakened, the balance of the brow is changed, and it begins to lift naturally. Eyebrows return to their original position. It's a great operation, since it uses the body's own processes to put the brow in the right position.

Although there is a bit of excess skin when the operation is finished, there is no need to cut and sew it up. I merely staple the incision closed. The skin's natural elasticity is enough to assure that the needed contraction will occur.

When I'm done with the muscle work, I suspend the entire brow internally, and over the next six weeks it heals into place. Because I use absorbable sutures, there's nothing to remove at that point. At first, we used large sutures to put the brow back together, but we found that led to hair loss, so I developed a system for a tunnel and a suture that holds everything together internally. That technique evolved into a biodegradable self-absorbing suspension device, and that's the system that I patented. It's one of my proudest achievements as a doctor.

And I owe it all to a bunch of deadheads.

The Eyes Have It—Eye Jobs

Eye complaints are incredibly common, and eye surgery can be incredibly successful, with minimal pain and risks.

As long as it's done properly.

When someone is looking directly at you, you shouldn't see any skin overhanging the upper lid. There should be a well-defined fold, with a specific natural curve. Lots of people have well-defined eyelids when they're younger. Then gravity takes over, and eyelids start to sag and droop, and people look either perpetually tired, or frustrated, or even angry. Getting rid of hooded eyes is the procedure known as upper blepharoplasty. If your problem is bags beneath your eye, you need a lower blepharoplasty.

We call them blephs.

Great progress has been made in eyelid surgery. (It's not eyeball surgery, so you don't have to worry about being blinded, unless something goes disastrously wrong in surgery.) In the old days—oh, I'd say maybe five years ago—we made the incision on the lower lid from below and removed what we thought was extra skin and fat. We didn't understand how delicate the eyelid is. A significant number of patients ended up with an ectropion, or a pulled-down lower lid that made them look like bloodhounds. It was a dead giveaway of an eyelid operation. Nobody was happy. We've learned our lesson, and the technique is refined enough so ectropions shouldn't happen.

When I mark up a patient before surgery with a pen so I'll know where to cut, I mark with the eye open and with the eye closed. When I was a plastic surgery fellow I was taught to pick up the skin, but I soon realized that wasn't a good idea—it doesn't put the eye in a natural state. You get an artificial-looking result if you distort the skin when you're making the scalpel marks. The most important thing is to leave enough skin in the lid so that the eye will close postoperatively.

That sounds obvious, and yet it's a deformity that is too often inflicted on people. Lots of doctors are now advertising their skill with blephs. Doctors who take short courses on eyelid surgery may think they're simple procedures, but trust me, they aren't. They're not nearly as complicated as face-lifts, but they need a deft touch. When the incision to take out fat or excess skin is not made properly, a notch can be left on the upper eyelid. When too much skin is taken out of the lid, you can't close your eye completely. Or you get the dreaded ectropion when too much is taken out below the eye, and the lower lid sags as a result.

When that happens, I can try to fix it by doing a canthopexy, which involves tightening the ligament of the lower eyelid. Of course, the key is to avoid getting into that position in the first place. Be sure to ask your surgeon how many eye procedures he or she has done and how he or she was trained.

If the doctor waffles, put on your sunglasses and head for the door.

Another thing. If you have lines between your eyebrows but a properly placed brow, surgery is too extreme. Giving a patient a brow-lift for worry lines or wrinkles is like taking a shotgun to kill a fly. Don't let anyone talk you into it. Botox is a perfect solution until a brow-lift is really necessary.

And the Winner . . . by a Nose—Rhinoplasty

Rhinoplasty may be one of the most commonly performed facial procedures, but patients still end up getting nervous about their nose jobs. That's hardly surprising. Getting rid of a really big nose can become a really big deal. The entire look of the face can immediately and sometimes irrevocably be changed by fiddling with the nose, and if you don't know what you're doing, you can change a face for the worse. In addition, patients worry that their nose will end up being crooked, or tipped up, or pinched in, or that they won't be able to breathe.

Whether I am smoothing out a bump in a nose or slimming an overly wide one, I use the same procedure. It's called an open rhinoplasty. It involves more time, but I think it produces a better result because it gives me more control.

I start by making an incision at the base of the nose and then lifting up most of the skin. I cut the cartilage and file the bone to make it smaller, smooth out any hump, then work on the cartilage structure in the middle of the nose. I have to break the nose to realign the nasal bones, to straighten it out, or to narrow it.

That's why you end up looking like you've been knocked out in the ring after a nose job. It isn't a dainty procedure.

The most delicate part of the work involves the tip of the nose. Many people, as they age, find that the tip starts to hang down unattractively. To lift it back up again, I often support it with what's called a cartilage graft. I take cartilage from a different part of the nose, or even from the ear, and use it to prop up the tip, the way the base of an umbrella holds up the nylon that keeps you dry.

Nose jobs aren't easy, and I see a lot of other people's mistakes. I worked on a woman who'd had five surgeries done on her nose. She had been in a snowmobile accident and had badly broken her nose. Doctor after doctor tried unsuccessfully to correct it. By the time she got to me, her nose looked flat. I had to slim it down *and* build it up. It was a very long operation.

Some doctors take out too much cartilage or bone, or they end up making the nose asymmetrical. I think that happens because most doctors use a procedure called the closed rhinoplasty. In that process, the incisions are made inside. Those doctors are looking underneath the skin and just hoping that they're removing the right amount of bone and cartilage. Dissection in an open rhinoplasty is more complex, but it provides for an unbeatable level of accuracy.

Let's Face It—Face-Lifts

Eventually, Botox isn't enough.

Sometime in their forties or their fifties, people tend to look in the mirror and not recognize the person who is looking back. Or they stop looking altogether. Because it's no joy to see deep lines between the nose and mouth, creases on the forehead, a badly drooping jawline, and a saggy neck. No injectible can take care of all of those problems. Besides, going for injections every six months gets to be awfully expensive and time-consuming. Especially when I can tighten the underlying muscles, redrape the skin over them, and move the malar fat pads, which form the lines from the nose to the mouth, back up to their original position to reduce the nasolabial fold. A face-lift gets things over with once and for all.

A face-lift can work wonders—if you go to the right surgeon. But if you go to a surgeon who's not very good, lots of damage can be done— drooping eyebrows, skin pulled incorrectly, or worst of all, permanent nerve damage that can leave you unable to smile, have a natural expression, raise your eyebrows, or even suck on a straw.

There are inherent risks to any surgical procedure with even the most expert doctor. You can get an infection, or there can be an unexpected reaction to the anesthesia. The likelihood of problems is slim, but the risks exist. Patients, of course, never want to believe they can happen to them. Until they happen.

There is no such thing as one procedure fits all when it comes to face-lifts. Doctors trying to get an edge in this business boast that they have perfected the short scar face-lift, or the minilift, or the lunch hour lift, but we all have pretty much the same techniques at our disposal. The more work the face needs, the longer the incision will have to be. But figuring out exactly what a face needs is not easy. That's where my aesthetic judgment comes into play. The initial consultation isn't just an opportunity for potential patients to ask questions. It's a deep visual examination, and the conclusions I make are crucial in determining what technique to use.

During surgery, a doctor who doesn't pull the skin hard enough will get a look that is less appealing than that achieved by a doctor who pulls it just right, and a doctor who pulls it too much will get the worst look of all. That's where you really see the differences among surgeons. When I first started out, I didn't pull the skin as tight as I do now. I learned over the years that it sags just a little bit after it heals, and I learned exactly how tight I could pull it without getting an unattractive scar or a too-tight look.

Patients, not surprisingly, don't really understand all of this. Why should they? It all boils down to trust. If they pick me, based on what I explain to them, based on previous photos, based on previous patients, they are giving me their trust that I will make their faces look younger, fresher, and more natural—and not pulled so much and so distorted that they look like they'd just stepped out of a wind tunnel.

When patients come in for an initial consultation, I hold up a mirror and say, "Tell me what you see. Tell me what you don't like." I listen carefully. Then I tell them whether I can change what they don't like, and if so, how it would be done.

My Typical Face-Lift Ladies

Simone was fifty-eight and her sister Carrie was fifty-six. They were charming, well educated, funny, articulate women who came in one day, eager to talk about what I could do for them.

"I'm here because I want some nips and tucks," said Simone. "I'm starting to look more tired. Even though I'm in good health, thank goodness, and I exercise all the time, and I don't smoke. The only medication I take is an antidepressant."

I asked her to close her eyes and relax her forehead. The room was silent for a few minutes as I intently studied her face.

The first thing I try to figure out is whether the eyelids are hanging over the eyes too much because they have excess skin and fat, or because the brow has dropped, or for both reasons. That's a very important distinction and decision. If I believe the problem is the eyelid, and I take out excess skin and fat, the problem will not be wholly solved if in fact the brow was descending, thanks to gravity.

Next I look at the lower two-thirds of the face, which is the section that falls under the category of a face-lift.

"You do have a fair amount of skin on your upper eyelids, but your brow has descended a little bit," I told her. I lifted up her eyebrows slightly with my hand. "When I do this, it doesn't completely eliminate the excess skin, but it gets rid of the hooding. That tells me that you have a malposition of the brow. An endoscopic brow-lift is the perfect solution."

I explained the procedure to her. "The other big benefit to the endoscopic brow-lift is that you don't get that surprised look people used to have with a brow-lift, with their eyebrows unnaturally lifted up."

At the same time, I told her, I would trim the excess skin of the upper eyelids, putting an elliptical incision in the creases. "Because it's placed in a natural crease, the scar heals incredibly well. That's really the secret to getting good scars—place them properly. And on your lower eyelids, it's only a matter of excess fat. Most people tend to have some there—it has nothing to do with how much you eat. Plus your skin is good. The way I address that is from the inside of the lid and just take out the fat."

Simone sat pondering. She'd obviously come in thinking she needed just a little skin taken off of her eyelids, not an entire forehead adjustment.

"If I removed only the skin on the upper eyelid," I said, "you would be happy for a few months, and then you'd start to get unhappy. Six months after that, your brow would have descended even farther, and the problem would not have been solved."

I continued analyzing her face.

"As for your face and neck," I went on, "if you wanted to eliminate your jowls and the skin and fat hanging beneath your chin, the incision would start in the temple and then go inside of the ear, a placement called the retrotragal incision. Ten years ago, the incisions were much more visible because they went in front of the ear. Now, after going inside the ear, the incision goes around the earlobe in the crease and into the hairline, not along the hairline. Because of that route, it's now possible to wear your hair up or very short after a face-lift. If somebody actually looks behind your ear, all he or she will see is a fine white line."

"That's good," she murmured, and her sister nodded.

Then I told her how I'd do aggressive liposuction in the neck, lift up her malar fat pads to smooth out the lines between her nose and her mouth, tighten the muscles, redrape her skin, and cut off any excess.

Unlike many of my patients, Simone and Carrie didn't blanch at my fairly graphic description. They were really paying attention. I knew they'd be terrific patients.

"What about anesthesia?" Simone asked.

"For someone of your age and state of excellent health, you only need twilight sleep, not general anesthesia," I replied. "The anesthesiologist uses a drug called propofol. I think it's safer. You're breathing on your own. The respiratory center is not suppressed. And because the drug is lighter, recovery is much quicker. In less than two hours, sometimes less than an hour after the conclusion of the surgery, you'll be awake. There is far less tendency for nausea and vomiting than with general anesthesia, but to reduce the chances even further, I give my patients an antinausea medication before the surgery.

"Yesterday," I went on, "a patient went home from here an hour and a half after surgery. When I trained, patients like you would have been admitted to a hospital for two or three days. Not because of the surgery, but because of the anesthesia." A nurse, I told her, would have to go home with her the first night to check her blood pressure and to make sure she wasn't developing a hematoma, which is a collection of fluid under the skin.

Any severe problems usually happen in the first eight hours after surgery. The next morning, she would return to the office, and I would take out the drains that were moving fluid out of her face and wrap her in a small bandage. She would be all set.

I told her that the complication rate in such a procedure is very small, but that I could never say it was zero. The overall complication rate in aesthetic surgery was less than one percent. The recovery would move quickly in the beginning and then slow down. After two weeks she could easily go out in public. For six weeks, she wouldn't look her very best. But then, voilà, she'd look terrific—like herself but with a natural change. Not an unnatural one.

"What I want you to come back and say is, 'My friends tell me I look better, but they don't know exactly why,'" I said.

"Right," she said. "They'll ask me if I lost weight."

"If I do my job correctly—and I will—no one should look at you and automatically be able to assume you've had a face-lift."

"That's always been my biggest fear about a face-lift," she admitted. "My daughter walks down the street with me and points at some overstretched woman, and then she says, 'Mom, you don't want a face-lift. Look at *her*.'"

"Don't worry. I'm not likely to do that. If you're not completely happy with how you look, and feel like you need any revisions, I'll do them for you. As long as I agree that it makes sense aesthetically and is feasible. On every patient, I keep going until I achieve the best result I can. If there's a problem, I take care of you."

"Great."

"My turn now," said Carrie good-naturedly, giving her sister a shove out of the way. They laughed. "So take a good look," she went on. "About six years ago, I had a double mastectomy, and since I was going through all that hell, I gave myself a treat and had my eyes done and a face-lift too. But I don't think that doctor did a very good job. Look, you can see the scar on my ear. Can you fix it?"

I examined it and told her that I could move the incision farther back.

"That's just what I wanted to hear," she said, sighing in relief. "And what can you do about the rest of my face? I'm getting bags under my eyes again, and there are so many lines around my mouth too. And my chin is all floppy and drooping. I look like a hound dog."

"I wouldn't go that far," I said with a smile. "Unfortunately, it's inevitable that your skin continues to age after surgery, in part due to sun exposure and in part due to natural processes. Not every face-lift starts to fall in six years, but some do. Most last at least twelve to fifteen years. You'll continue to age, of course, but twenty years down the line, you'll still be a lot better off than if you hadn't had any work done at all."

Then I looked at the skin under her eyes. "I think a laser can help with the crepey nature of your skin here, as well as with your crow's-feet. The laser I use is very effective, but in some ways it's harder to recover from than the face-lift. It's a second-degree burn, going into the midlayer of the dermis. The collagen bundles there contract, the skin tightens, and the superficial lines disappear. For five days or so it's an open wound that just sort of weeps. You keep washing it and putting ointment on it. After five days of looking pretty scary, new skin forms, and it has that pink look of fresh skin, the way your knee looked when you fell off your bicycle as a kid and skinned it. For six months or so, you might need to wear makeup, until the lasered skin matches the surrounding skin.

"It's a process," I added. "It takes patience. And I would be lying to you if I said that it was completely pain free. You'll have a burning sensation for about twenty-four hours. You put ice compresses on it, and we give you pain medication to control it. There's also a chance with laser of the skin becoming hyperpigmented, meaning darker. If it did, bleaching creams could lessen the effect. But there's also a chance that the skin could become hypopigmented, meaning lighter. If that happened, it would be permanent and there would be nothing that could be done to fix it. That patch of skin would require makeup all the time. There's no way of predicting," I said. "You have light eyes and fair skin, so it's less likely."

"Is that how you would also treat the lines around the mouth?" she asked.

"Yes."

"Oh, I'll be really attractive coming out of this one," she said.

"I know. Just don't plan any parties." I smiled. "I've worked with chemical peels and dermabrasion, but laser really is the best approach because it goes deeper and it's longer lasting. With dermabrasion, a spinning wire brush quickly scrapes the skin, but it's difficult to control, and the results aren't as dramatic. Laser is the most controlled way of wounding the skin," I told her. "Hopefully, a laser will soon be invented that'll tighten the skin without burning it. Once that happens, who needs a scalpel?"

"Call me the minute that happens," Carrie said with a laugh. "And it better be before I kick the bucket!"

Ladies of a Certain Age

Occasionally I see older patients, the kind of women who used to make up the bulk of my practice. Nancy was seventy-two years old and in good health. As always, I asked her what was bothering her.

"I don't know what I need done," she said. "I just want to look neat."

I asked her if what mostly bothered her was her neck, because it was extremely crepey and sagging.

"No, not really. It's my eyes and around my mouth. My neck doesn't bother me quite as much."

"Do you smoke?"

"Not anymore. I was naughty, I know," she said. "We all smoked. Now I look at my wrinkles and wonder why I did it. Back then, who knew?"

"I know," I said. "Plus sun exposure is equally damaging. But no one talked about how bad that was, either."

"We loved to go to the beach and bask in the sun. No one had even heard of sunscreen."

"You're so right," I replied, then asked her to open her eyes and look at my nose without lifting her brow. "You have a lot of excess skin on your upper eyelids," I said after I examined her. "On your neck, you have these two prominent bands, called platysma bands, as well as a fair amount of excess skin. I would recommend a face-lift to improve your neck. And as for the wrinkles around your mouth, they can be improved only through laser resurfacing, which is effective but takes a long time to heal.

"It's real surgery," I went on. "You definitely have to have your internist give us clearance. I don't like surprises in the operating room." Her husband, who had been sitting silently reading a magazine, looked up at that point and expressed his approval for the idea of bringing in her regular doctor. "That's good advice," he said.

I told her that I had operated many times on people her age, but that certain procedures had to be followed. "A lot of plastic surgeons don't ask for medical clearances, but I do. I also ask smokers to stop lighting up at least two weeks before surgery and not to smoke for at least two weeks after surgery.

"Smokers simply do not do as well," I explained. "Their healing can be more difficult, especially their scars. It all has to do with the constriction of the blood vessels, which can affect their blood supply. Their skin flaps can turn terribly black and blue. Of course, a lot of smokers lie about quitting, because it's too difficult for them to do, and they tend to bleed more during surgery and have other complications. They also bruise more. It can really be a problem."

"I'm glad I quit already," Nancy said.

Her husband nodded again. "So am I," he said.

"It makes a real difference," I went on. "Many of my patients want to do well, so they use this time to stop smoking for good. My first priority is to make sure I don't do any harm to you. With all patients, we check their blood work and do a chest X-ray. And you'll have to have a stress test with your internist."

"Better to be safe than sorry," said her husband.

I also told her that because of her age, and because she was on blood pressure medication, she would have to have the surgery done in the hospital rather than the office, in case I needed to admit her. "After surgery, the worst thing you can do is go home and stay in bed. I want you to be active," I said. "The best thing you can do is walk."

The day after her surgery, which was pleasantly uneventful, Nancy came in to see me. I unwrapped her bandages and cleaned off her face. She looked awful, the way everyone looks the day after a face-lift. But it was clear that she was going to have a clean jawline for the first time in years, and a lovely neck. I took out the draining tubes and told her I would see her the next day.

"I'll just put an ace bandage on your neck and chin," I said. "You can take that off tomorrow morning and hop in the shower. If you must wash your hair, use only a gentle baby shampoo. No conditioner and no other hair products. Don't use a blow dryer, either, as the heat isn't good for you. Sleep on two pillows. No heavy lifting, please. And put Bacitracin on the incisions at least twice a day. It helps soften the scars, so they heal better. If you're in pain, take the pain medication as necessary. I don't want you to suffer. Please don't be afraid to take it."

I would see her again for a quick visit in three days, to check her progress.

When she came in, she was beaming. "I can't believe how much the swelling went down already," she said.

"It tends to go down very quickly at first," I explained. "But the very last tiny bit of swelling can take several months to disappear completely. It's a slow process."

But Nancy clearly didn't mind. She looked years younger, and she was thrilled.

The Young and the Beautiful

When Tina was a young model just starting out in New York, she came to me for collagen injections. Now she was thirty-eight, still modeling against all odds and wanting to keep getting jobs. She was not a happy camper about unavoidable signs of aging. If she didn't have a face-lift, she worried that she would soon lose her livelihood. Not surprisingly, the thought of tampering with her face, let alone having her surgery commented on publicly, terrified Tina.

And recently, she said, she had started seeing her father's face in the mirror.

"This part always bothered me," she said, placing her hand under her chin and stroking her nascent jowls as she sat in a consulting room. "I don't want to do anything drastic, but I'm starting to see my father's droopy jowls staring back at me whenever I look in the mirror. I can tell how it's all going to come crashing down here."

She was right. Although still a knockout, her inevitable facial sag was starting. For most people, I wouldn't recommend a face-lift at this point. But for models, their faces and their bodies *are* their work. Tina really didn't have much of a choice if she wanted to keep modeling.

"What's a minilift? Can I get one?" she asked.

"Sometimes it's called a short scar lift, and it's basically a standard face-lift that starts in the temple, goes inside of the ear, around the ear-lobe, and stops right behind the ear. The scar is smaller than it would be in an older patient who needs more skin removed," I replied. "For you, where you have only a little bit of extra skin in your neck, it's a good choice. It minimizes the incision, and the recovery time is shorter. I can't do it on a sixty-year-old with skin hanging down to here and jowls, but it does work well on people who want just a little bit done, most important with skin elastic enough to spring back. If done properly, no one will ever know you've had a face-lift. You'll look slightly different, fresher. Certainly not pulled or stretched."

"That's a relief." She managed a small smile.

"Typically, I do it here in the office under twilight sleep," I went on. "You don't need general anesthesia. I do recommend having a private duty nurse go home with you. Many of my patients stay at the Stan-hope Hotel, and then the next morning they come in and I take the dressings off. You should hide out for a week, because at first you'll look puffy, especially in your cheek area. After that, you can cover up any bruising with makeup. After a week, nobody will know. The scars typically heal very well. With your skin, you are prone to hypertrophic scars, which means they are raised, but it's very unlikely for that to happen on the face. I don't see that around the ear. The incisions are placed in the natural creases, and the chance of a hypertrophic scar is minimal.

"It's not very painful, but it's still surgery," I added, beginning the litany of side effects that I always explain to surgical patients. "The chance of infection is very rare. Hematoma is more likely in men and in those with high blood pressure. The worst risk was potential injury to the facial nerve."

Tina needed to fully understand all the risks, as slight as they were, because her face was central to her livelihood.

"Listen carefully. There are five nerve branches on each side of the face. I've been very lucky—in sixteen years I haven't had one instance of a nerve injury. But at the same time, that's the chance you take. To injure a nerve, I would have to be in the wrong level of dissection. If this happened and it was a permanent injury, you wouldn't be able to raise your eyebrow. Statistically, the chance of a nerve injury is less than one percent; out of that, twenty percent is permanent and eighty percent is temporary. So it's truly an almost infinitesimal risk. You know I have to tell you the truth, and the truth is that it's very unlikely to happen."

Tina smiled again. She didn't seem at all worried by the risk. She'd known me for a long time, she trusted me, and she didn't really consider that anything would go wrong. What she really wanted to know was what she would look like after the surgery.

"I'll give you a sense." I held up the mirror and pulled her skin just the slightest bit. "What I do is elevate this so it lessens your nasolabial fold. If you look at your kids, their malar fat pads are sitting up here." I placed my finger on the full part of the cheek. "That's where your malar fat pads are. They fall as we age. What I try to do is reposition them to lessen the indentation."

"But not pulled too far. Like Joan Rivers."

I laughed. "Everyone mentions her. No, not pulled too far. And certainly not like Joan Rivers. The likelihood of me doing that to you is zero, not only because I like you, but because I'd physically have to do things that I don't do during surgery. I'd have to pull the skin to the point where I would make an obvious, bad scar."

"No bad scars, please."

"Not to worry. And what about your upper eyelids?" I asked. "It's your call, but you might want a trim. Your brow is perfect. But there's just a little bit of excess skin in your upper lids. The incision is elliptical, right in your natural crease. It's very quick, a minor procedure. I put on a piece of steri strip and take it off after four days. At that point you can hardly see the incision."

"Sounds great. How long will all this last?"

"One out of five women will come back for a secondary face-lift. But most of them are much older than you. You'll still age but when you're fifty, you won't look fifty. Nothing will give you the fountain of youth. You'll still age."

"Tell me about it," she said ruefully. "Men can get older. Women can't. And you know what else—when I was younger my face was rounder. Now it looks longer."

I nodded. "That happens to everyone. As I said, the malar fat pads head south as we get older. Everything gets elongated."

"Where will my stitches be? I'm worried, because of the camera zooming in for close-ups."

"Inside and behind your ears. That's why this is such a cool operation. You can be in profile to the camera—it can even be right next to your face—and no lens will ever be able to pick up the incisions."

"That's a relief," she said and exhaled loudly. "I worked with some-one who had huge, horrible scars. He must've had his face-lift done years ago."

"He probably did. The problem with the old technique—and unfortu-nately, it still happens—is that the tension was placed on the skin. It was a skin-lift more than a face-lift. Anytime you close something under ten-sion, the skin eventually separates and creates a noticeable scar."

Tina nodded, then frowned. "Is this how I'll look?" she asked as she pulled her skin up a bit.

"Not quite." I moved her skin with my hand, to show her the proper angle of the lift. "Pull along this angle instead."

"So my face won't be flatter?"

"No."

"How bad will I look four days after the surgery?"

"You'll still be a little bit swollen, especially in your cheeks. Then the swelling will move down to the jowls, and then it disappears."

"Are people really not going to know that I did this?"

"They really shouldn't. If you don't want anybody to know, hide out for two weeks, not one."

"I'm pretty much going to look like me?"

"That's the key thing. I want people to say, 'You look great. You look well rested. Did you cut your hair?' Things like that. With your wonderful skin elasticity, this procedure really makes sense. And your eyes will heal very quickly. There's usually some black-and-blue bruising, but within ten days it goes away. After a week, you can go out and about with a pair of sunglasses and nobody will know that anything happened."

"So you definitely have no issues with me shooting a month after you do everything?"

"No. Not unless something unforeseen happens. Which, of course, shouldn't happen. Within a month, nobody will be able to see a thing."

"So you think this is a good thing for me?"

"I can't tell you that. I can only tell you the benefit of doing it now versus ten years from now," I gently explained. Tina's worries were perfectly understandable, and I was going to take all the time she needed to talk her through her anxiety. "I've taken care of a lot of patients in your business and I think I have a good sense of what you need to do for your job. So, yes, I think that you're right to do this. The rules that I apply to you may not apply to the woman who's sixty-five years old and whose closest link to the world of modeling is reading *Vogue*."

Tina laughed. "I also hate that my face is so lopsided. *This* profile is much nicer than *this* profile." She turned her face from side to side so I could see the difference. "When I'm on the right side of the camera, I look fatter and older."

"I agree," I said. "Don't hate me for saying that!"

I held up the mirror again and showed how I could compensate for her complaint. "We're all asymmetrical," I said. "There's nothing unusual about that. I wish I could just do liposuction on jowls, but I've seen too many problems with that. If a face-lift isn't also done, the skin will ripple and pucker over the area that had liposuction. It can look pretty awful."

"Will I actually feel tight after the surgery?"

"Initially, yes. You'll feel tight and swollen. It takes about six weeks to settle down. Most of the cheek swelling goes away in two or three days. Ninety percent is gone in a few weeks. So first you feel tight, and then everything relaxes."

Tina kept looking in the mirror, her face a mixture of fleeting emotions. I could feel her fear.

"Am I going to look like a freak?" she finally asked, almost sheepishly, knowing she had already asked that question ten different ways. But she knew I didn't mind her questions. She was thoughtful and careful.

As she should be.

"No. Within a week you can go out with friends. Your cheeks won't get black and blue, although in the neck it is possible."

"Maybe I'll do it in the winter. I can wear turtlenecks. I do feel like this is one thing I really want to do. I know you understand all the little nuances."

She told me about a fund-raiser coming up and asked if I'd be interested in going. I told her not to worry if she chose not to acknowledge me in public.

"Just last week," I explained, "I was having a drink at the Stanhope with Lorraine, waiting for some friends, when a patient of mine walked by with two others, who were also my patients. Not one said hello. Coincidentally, the husband of one came in the next day for a follow-up, and he apologized with a laugh. I told him it never bothers me to be snubbed. It goes with the territory."

"Speaking of the Stanhope," she said, "I guess I should stay there. I don't want my husband or kids to see me looking beat up. Besides, my husband is totally against this. I'll probably have to lie a little bit." She giggled. "I'm sure you've been in this situation before."

"Many times. Wives tell their husbands that they've just had a little fat taken out from beneath their eyes when in fact they had a full face-lift. Or when they have injectibles and they get swollen, they tell them that they were in the back of a cab and it stopped short and threw them against the divider. That's the perfect New York excuse. Another one is to say that they've had dental work when in fact they've had Botox. My favorite was the patient whose arms I did. She slept in long-sleeved pajamas for about six weeks because she didn't want her husband to know she had had surgery. It's totally understandable. What do you think you'll tell your husband?"

"I don't know yet. I did tell him I had an appointment, but only to talk about Botox and things like that. He has great respect for you."

"That's good. Just minimize it."

"I think I'll tell him that for the camera I need to get some fat off."

"It's not a bad idea for you to be away from home for a couple of days."

"Okay. Sign me up. Let's get this over with. I'll stay at the Stanhope." Then she winked. "But I better warn you—you may have to testify in my divorce."

Tina's surgery was a breeze. She healed like a dream. She was extremely happy with her improved face and eyes.

And I didn't have to testify in her divorce. Her husband still doesn't know she had a face-lift, and she has no plans to tell him.

Twelve

NEVER HAPPY: BREAST WORK

BREASTS COME IN ALL SHAPES AND ALL SIZES. UNFORTUNATELY, ALL THESE shapes and sizes often end up on the wrong bodies. Petite women can be burdened with disproportionately large breasts, which cause them years of debilitating back and shoulder pain, to say nothing of the embarrassment they deal with every day from callous and stupid strangers staring at their chests. Women with large breasts often feel they can't ever be taken seriously in the workplace, as their busts literally get in the way.

Women with small breasts, on the other hand, often spend much of their adult life wondering why they've been shortchanged in the femininity department. They can feel like perpetual teenagers, waiting, as one patient so succinctly put it, "to sprout."

And then there's Hollywood. I read an article in *US* magazine last year, where the actress Debra Messing, who is very small breasted, confessed, "When I first came to Hollywood, I was told that to achieve success as an actress you simply must have implants. Well, I didn't want to go that route. I thought I looked just fine."

Too many actresses don't have her resolve. And too many actresses have misshapen breasts as a result.

Most patients seeking breast work come for breast augmentation, which is not as complicated and major a procedure as breast reduction. Some come for a breast-lift, especially after weight loss or breast-feeding, and they often decide to add implants at the same time. They tend to be in their early or midthirties, finished with having their babies and eager to regain their old bodies. Although there are exceptions, they are not in the least embarrassed. They fling off their clothes and get right to their questions about breast size and shape.

Most of them just want modestly larger breasts—no over-the-top, Hollywood-ludicrous golden globes for these women. And they understand that it is a slightly longer recuperation time to have the implants put under, rather than over, the muscle.

Plenty of doctors take shortcuts on breast implants. And I have to say, the only good thing about a botched breast implant is that it can be removed.

Here's what can go wrong with breasts implants.

- It's rare, but implants can deflate or rupture. Twice I've seen them deflate when the scar tissue grows into the valve and lifts it open. Rupture happens with trauma. One patient went rock climbing, and the partner who was securing her fell on top of her and ruptured both implants. She went to the hospital to treat the bruises and contusions on her face and the rest of her body, and then came into my office afterward. Unfortunately, her implants had to be replaced, but she came through without any permanent damage or scarring. This gives you some idea of the amount of force it takes to damage an implant. Sex definitely won't rupture them.
- The body naturally forms scar tissue around the implant, which is to be expected. This is no big deal unless an inordinate amount of scar forms. In that case, it is called a capsule, and it can look and feel awkward, so it has to be cut out. The implant is exchanged and the capsule resected to make the breast soft again.

- Most problems I see are caused by doctors misusing their scalpels. If the implant is inserted *above* the muscle, it can move. That's right—a migrating implant. It can inch up so that it rests above where it ought to be—and where it ought to be is in your breast, not above it.

  Some doctors, on the other hand, manage to put the implants in too low, so that you have two hanging spheres. Recently I saw a very pretty thirty-six-year-old woman with a perfect body— except for her breasts. Her implants were sitting so low it looked as if she had two rocks in a sock hanging from each side of her chest. This was not a problem with implants—it was a problem with her surgeon's judgment. The implants had been placed in the wrong plane, above the muscle, as well as placed too low.

Although I have my doubts that silicone gel caused the problems that some women believed it caused, I don't see any need at this point for silicone gel implants. There was a large, rigorously controlled study that showed no cause and effect between silicone implants and cancer, lupus, or anything else. In my opinion, that issue has been put to bed. Still, I agree with the FDA that more longitudinal studies are needed to show that there are no diseases that result from the silicone gel implants. A longer period of tracking patients would answer all the questions. The implants I use are silicone bags with saline inside.

During consultations, patients who have not had children sometimes ask whether they will able to breast-feed if they have implants. Routinely, they will, but I tell them that if they absolutely want a guarantee about breast-feeding, they should hold off on the implants. Although the risk is slight, there could be a situation where the implant would make it impossible to breast-feed—from a hematoma, for instance, or scarring. When in doubt, it's always best not to proceed.

Let's take a look at three patients who had different breast procedures.

Margaret: A Little Cleavage Would Be Nice

Margaret was thirty-two, trim and toned, about five-seven, and had a successful career as a software designer.

"Software is what I've got down there," she joked about her breasts. "I kept thinking they would grow when I got older. And they didn't. So here I am."

Margaret was barely a B cup, and having her breasts augmented would give her the cleavage she'd wanted for years.

The most important question I asked her had to do with her family history. I asked whether there was a strong family history of breast cancer, meaning that either her mother or her sister had it. The reason for this is not that implants cause cancer—just the opposite. A study showed that there was a greater likelihood that cancer would be detected earlier in women with implants. The explanation was simple. Those women are told to go for a mammogram every year, which they might not have done if they hadn't had the implants. A mammogram is essential prior to implant surgery, because scar tissue around the implants can make it difficult to get a good picture during future mammograms. Only nine percent of the cases get so much scar tissue that a mammogram becomes compromised, but in a woman with a strong breast cancer risk, that's just too high a probability. So if Margaret had had a strong family history, I simply would have told her that a breast implant was too risky for her.

One of the most important things I do is customize the surgery to the patient. I get the feeling sometimes that if you go to some other states, surgeons just line the patients up and give them all exactly the same thing, and boom, after a couple of cases, the doctor has covered his or her monthly overhead.

I'm lucky, because thankfully I can afford to do what's best for the patient. Margaret's surgery went well, and it was typical of the breast augmentations I do. I make an incision in the inframammary fold, which is just under the breast, cut down to the pectoralis major muscle, and develop a pocket underneath the muscle. After I make sure there is no bleeding, I put the implant in. In some cases, I go through the areola instead, but it depends on which approach will work best for the patient in terms of scarring.

Then, while Margaret was still asleep on the table in the operating room, I asked Lolita and Tim to sit her up, so that I could see how the larger breast looked. It still seemed to me a bit too small, considering her build, so I had them put her back down. Then I added some saline to the implant. Each implant has a port in the front, which makes it easy to add or take out however much saline solution is necessary to get the right look. That's a huge advantage over the old silicone gel implants, which came in set sizes.

Then I had them sit her up again. This time, I liked what I saw. This is the artistic part of the job, and there's just no way to explain how I do it. It's about having a sense of proportion, of balance. Because I was satisfied that the breasts perfectly suited her body, I sewed up the incision.

Margaret came in about five days later, saying that it hurt quite a bit more than she expected. That's because I cut her muscle, and cutting muscle hurts. There is simply no way around it. I told her that by the end of the week she could do anything she wanted to do, except heavy lifting. And of course she had already gone back to work. The surgery required her to take only a few days off.

At her last follow-up appointment, Margaret was delighted. Her pain had soon subsided. "I've already bought three new bikinis," she said. "And I'm finally going to fill them out!"

Pamela: The Curse of the Large Breasts

Big breasts can be a curse.

Forty-year-old Pamela sat in my office, wiping away tears. "I don't just want to get rid of these things," she said, pointing to her chest. "I *need* to get rid of them. My neck and back have been killing me for years, and they're compounding my arthritis. You've got to help me."

"What size bra do you wear?" I asked.

"I'm not sure," she replied. "I have to have them custom-made."

I took a tape measure from the drawer and asked her to open her gown. I stretched the tape from her collarbone to the center of her nipple. When breasts are of average size and they haven't sagged, that number tends to be nineteen or twenty centimeters. In her case, it was thirty-five centimeters.

"Not that there's an ideal measurement," I said, "but it should probably be in the twenty-centimeter range." I explained that breast reduction is major surgery, done under general anesthesia, and that it could take a long time, up to two and a half hours. If not done correctly, it can put the blood supply to the nipple at risk. Nor is liposuction of the breasts an option. Tissue and fat must be cut out, and the breasts have to be remolded. Even when they have to live with chronic pain, women tend to think about the implications of breast reduction for a long time before they finally go ahead, because it can be a drastic change.

"Your nipples will move up a great deal, from somewhere near your waist to a point midway down your upper arm," I told Pamela. "Because you have fair skin, your scars should heal very well. Eventually, you'll have only tiny white lines on your breast, in the shape of an inverted T, like the incision."

"Will I still be able to feel anything in my nipples?" she asked.

"That's what I always strive for," I replied. "I do everything possible to maintain feeling in the nipple, but there's always a chance in such a large reduction that there would be compromising of the blood supply and that I would have to then use a technique called the 'free nipple graft.' It's a radical approach, so I never start off thinking I need to use it, but it's good to know the technique is there if it is required."

"What do you mean?"

"A 'free nipple graft' technique involves the complete removal of the nipple and creating a new one, which may not have the same appearance or sensation. I've never had to do that, so don't even think about it. It's no cause for worry.

"Don't focus on that," I told her. "That's a very radical approach. But due to your age and the various medications you take already, I'll have to do the surgery in the hospital. You'll be sore for a few days, but the pain shouldn't be excruciating."

"I live with excruciating pain every day already," she said. "I'm not afraid of that!"

"Sounds like you're ready to go. We'll have one more consultation before your surgery, so think of any questions you have and I'll be glad to answer them." Then I told her what I always told breast reduction patients: the possible risks. These included infection; a hematoma, which is a pooling of blood under the skin; bad scarring; and lack of sensation in the nipples. "After the surgery is completed, I'll put drains underneath your breasts; I'll take them out the next morning. Then you'll need a simple dressing over your stitches, and you'll be able to wear any bra without an underwire, like a sports bra. You won't be able to do any exercise for several weeks."

I have seen few people look happier at the thought of surgery.

"Oh, it's going to be so wonderful. You have no idea. I can't wait to walk around without pain. And I can't wait to buy some new clothes that aren't baggy on top!"

"Wait awhile before buying a new wardrobe," I said with a laugh. "It takes a while for the swelling to go down. You won't know the true size of your breasts until at least a month after surgery."

"Whatever size they're going to be," she said, her smile wide, "they're going to be better than this!"

Jessica: Lift and Separate

Jessica was thrilled with her new weight: 135 pounds on her five-foot-six frame. She'd lost more than a hundred pounds after two years of following a low-carb diet combined with a rigorous workout regimen, and she was a woman transformed at thirty-eight.

Her breasts, however, were transformed too. They were not particularly large, but they sagged so badly that her nipples nearly reached to her waist.

"You're an ideal candidate for a breast-lift," I told her. "And it's fairly simple. It involves tightening the skin so that the breast returns to its original position. There is no muscle work, and as a result, not much pain. Do you have any questions?"

"I have sort of an embarrassing question," she replied. "About my nipples. One of my friends who had a breast-lift told me that her nipples aren't as sensitive anymore, and they never become erect."

"That's a good question," I told her, "because it is true that in some breast surgeries, reduced nipple sensation can result. But I use what's called the inferior pedicle technique. I don't interfere with any of the tissue directly under the nipple, so I don't compromise the nerves or the blood supply. And because a breast-lift is far less extensive than a breast reduction, I'm much less likely to have to alter the nipple. If it's handled well, you should maintain sensation in the nipples."

Her face brightened. "That's a relief. And what about working out? I need to stick to my routine, you know. It's a really important part of my life."

"You can start a light exercise routine after two weeks—get on a stationary bike or walk on a high-incline treadmill, something like that. But you will need to avoid lifting heavy weights for at least a month. You can otherwise resume all normal activities."

"Am I going to need a special bra after surgery?"

"Once the bandages come off, five to seven days after surgery, a sports bra will be fine, as long as it doesn't have an underwire in it."

"I've sure got plenty of those," she said. "I can't wait to get this over with!"

After the surgery, she came in for the usual postoperative checkup, and she looked wonderful. But she had one question about something that was really worrying her.

"My breasts look great, but there's a wrinkle on each one," she said. "What is that from? Will it go away?"

"It takes usually six months for everything to be completely normal. And you are more swollen on your right side than your left. After all, I moved your breasts a long, long way to get them back to their correct position."

"I bet you did," she said. "Probably about a foot."

I laughed. "Well, it was more like a half a foot. Eventually, everything will settle down and the wrinkles will go away."

"And then you can take care of the wrinkles on my face," she said happily.

Thirteen

LIPOSUCTION AND TUMMY TUCKS: SAY GOOD-BYE TO THUNDER THIGHS AND TREMBLING TUMMIES

THERE'S A LOT OF FAT OUT THERE.

The most popular surgical procedure practiced by plastic surgeons in America right now is liposuction. There were an estimated three hundred thousand liposuctions done in 2003, and the figure is expected to keep rising. Not surprisingly, I tend to get more liposuction patients in Santa Rosa, in northern California's beautiful wine country, where I work one week out of every six with my twin brother, Marek, the dermatologist. It makes sense. People are usually more body conscious when they live in an environment with pleasant weather, where their legs and arms are exposed frequently.

But the patients I see in New York are pretty body conscious too.

Liposuction has revolutionized our profession, because it's not regular cut-and-stitch surgery. In the old days, if you wanted your thighs and arms thinner, we had to cut out skin and fat, and the resulting incision left a long, unattractive scar. Liposuction allows for body sculpting with almost no scarring. It is, however, a far less exact procedure than a face-lift, because the scalpel is more controllable than a cannula and a suction machine. Plus patients don't need general anesthesia, only twilight sleep.

The anesthesia is so quickly metabolized that the patient wakes up in a half hour or forty-five minutes after the procedure.

Before you're out, when you're standing up, I mark the places where I plan to pull out fat. Then, when you lie down, I see how your skin falls into various positions. Even with the marks I make, liposuction is a far less exact procedure than other surgeries because the solution I inject slightly distorts the skin. I inject a combination of lidocaine and epinephrine to cut down on bleeding and to minimize postoperative pain. The anesthesiologist also puts fluid back into the body through an IV line, to compensate for the amount that will be removed when a combination of fluid, fat, and blood is pulled out during the liposuction process. The sum of what I infiltrate, plus what the anesthesiologist gives, should be equal to the amount that I remove. That just seems to work hemodynamically. Essentially, liposuction is a process that is all about maintaining a healthy balance in the body as fluids are removed.

Some surgeons claim that best results occur when the patient is standing up during liposuction. I disagree. Unless you are doing just the tiniest bit of liposuction, I think that's dangerous. The patient is unstable and could pass out. In the worst-case scenario, you could even kill someone by having him or her stand up in that state, because the blood pressure could suddenly crash.

Overall, though, liposuction is a great procedure, and I fully understand its popularity. As long as reasonable amounts of fat are removed during liposuction, it is safe, and recovery is relatively fast. For more significant drooping skin and fat in the belly, the tummy tuck, or abdominoplasty, is the procedure of choice.

The key is patient selection, knowing which procedure is appropriate. Although many women come to me hoping for a shortcut, liposuction should not be used instead of a diet. It's not to be thought of cavalierly as an instant way to lose weight. It works best for women who have specific areas of fat deposits around their thighs, hips, or bellies that they just can't shed, no matter how much they exercise and maintain a normal weight. And it's a godsend for men who have excess fat in their breast area, a condition known as gynecomastia. These men are usually mortified by what looks like breasts and ecstatic when it can be fixed, which I discuss in the next chapter.

Although it's crucial to take out only small amounts of fat, there are doctors who push the envelope and run into trouble. Massive liposuction really pisses me off. It's irresponsible. It's risky. And I don't know why anyone does it.

Because it can be lethal.

Fat contains a lot of liquid and some blood, which is removed during liposuction. Take out too much fluid, and you destabilize the body's delicate balance. As I've said, fluid is also injected during liposuction, and that too, if not handled properly, can result in an imbalance.

It's hard to say how risky liposuction is, because many states don't require doctors to report cases with negative consequences. Although I've seen estimates that suggest there are three deaths for every hundred thousand procedures—which is three too many—a worrisome survey of twelve hundred members of the American Society of Plastic Surgeons, which appeared in the journal *Plastic and Reconstructive Surgery,* found a higher death rate. The generally accepted mortality rate for elective surgery is one in fifty thousand. More studies are being done to try to figure out if those numbers are correct, but at the very least, they point out the need for caution.

The study found that the most frequent cause of death during liposuction was a pulmonary embolism, created when a blood clot or fat entered and damaged the lungs. Other fatal complications included perforations of the abdominal wall, anesthesia problems, and respiratory failure. The death rate was much higher when liposuction was combined with other surgical procedures.

Unless there is an unavoidable disaster like an allergic reaction, no one should ever be at risk from liposuction due to a doctor's incompetence— or arrogance.

One plastic surgeon in New York claims that we can safely take out up to twenty pounds of fat during liposuction. She argues that being overweight presents a greater long-term risk than the risk posed by the liposuction. I don't believe that, mainly because you can kill someone getting her there. I don't want to be lumped in with this plastic surgeon; to me, she's providing nothing more than a disservice to our profession. New York University has guidelines for liposuction that suggest taking out no more than ten pounds of fat, and that is considered the ultimate top, which should be done only in a hospital. I think it's crazy to take more than that.

Liposuction seekers, beware! Find a good doctor who doesn't promise to suck out more than ten pounds of fat at one time. Any doctor who does that is just sucking out your bank account and risking your health.

Amanda, a fit woman of fifty-four, knew that. She was a typical liposuction patient.

"I'm not just losing all the skirmishes—I'm losing the battle too," she said. "I can't seem to get rid of my stomach. Menopause sucks. I've noticed that my stomach has been getting looser in the last year or so. I managed to keep it together for a long time, and now this!"

I examined her abdomen closely.

"Actually, I think it's more from pregnancy than menopause," I told her. "What you have is very typical. The fascia, which is the covering of the muscle, gets stretched. Once you stretch it, you can do a million sit-ups and it won't make any difference."

"I could have told you that," she said with a wry smile. "I've been going to the gym three days a week for years. You'd think it would make a dent."

"It does make a dent," I replied. "It's obvious how well toned you are. But even if your muscles are strong, the fascia is not part of that."

"So can liposuction help me?"

"It can, but it won't take care of everything that is bothering you. The only way to give you an absolutely flat stomach is an abdominoplasty, or tummy tuck," I told her. "But I wouldn't recommend a tummy tuck for you. It would be overkill. You really don't have that much excess skin. Plus your skin's elasticity is pretty good. That's what makes you an ideal candidate for liposuction."

Liposuction permanently removes fat cells. Once they are gone, they can't come back. If you happen to gain weight—and some of my patients do—it should be evenly distributed over the rest of the body.

"In doing liposuction of the belly," I told Amanda, "I numb the area and then use a cannula, or metal tube, to go through an incision and into the layer of fat. I use an ultrasonic technique that breaks up the fat, which makes it easier to take out. A machine that's like a vacuum cleaner sucks out the fat from the body through the cannula. What comes out is a yellowish fluid, tinted slightly pink from blood.

"You can go home within an hour or an hour and a half. You'll feel sore, as if you'd had a vigorous workout, but the pain is easily manageable. There's very little blood loss, but you'll get black and blue.

"There are possible complications," I added. "When I push the cannula through your fat cells, I create little tunnels. They can fill up with fluid. That is very infrequent, but it can happen. If it does, I have to drain them."

"Does that hurt?" she asked. "Will I look hideous?"

"It is a fairly rare occurrence," I said, "so don't worry about it. If I did have to drain the fluid, I would just take it out with a needle and a syringe.

"There is also the possibility of indentations or irregularities in the skin," I went on. "Someone with poor skin elasticity is more likely to have irregularities. After surgery, you'll need to wear an elastic compression garment, like a girdle, to keep down the swelling. It's a must to use it.

"After forty-eight hours, it's a good idea to have a Jacuzzi. Your muscles will feel very sore, and that warmth helps relax them. Some people still feel pretty awful, and in that case I can prescribe Valium, which is a muscle relaxant."

"When can I go back to work?" she wondered.

"I've had patients go back to work the same day, but I think that's insane." I smiled and shook my head. "They didn't want to listen. I think you should take a couple of days off, drink a lot of fluids, and go home and put pillows under your knees and relax. Take it easy. Your body needs to recuperate."

"How long before I see real changes?"

"The first time you take off the compression garment, you'll look down there and say, 'What's going on here? He didn't do anything.' That's due to the swelling. By six weeks, you'll see a significant change. Still, it can take up to six months for all of the scarring to go away and for your skin to feel normal to the touch."

"Yikes! That long?"

"It's not so bad, really. You ought to be very happy after six weeks."

"Well, I've lived with this belly for so long, I guess a few more weeks won't hurt!" Amanda said and went to see Lorraine to book the procedure.

Another patient, Kate, was also an ideal candidate for liposuction. At thirty-seven, she consistently did Pilates and had a perfectly flat stomach to show for all her hard work. Her thighs, though, drove her crazy.

"Look at this," she said, grabbing them on the outside. "I try and try and try, and nothing makes them look better."

"Fat deposits on your lateral thighs are incredibly common," I told her. "This is by far the most common area of liposuction women need. It's perfectly normal to have excess fat there."

"It's perfectly *gross*," she said with a laugh.

"If it makes you feel any better, I've operated on marathon runners who don't have an ounce of fat except for their lateral thighs," I replied. "No amount of exercise can change the actual shape of your thighs or remove that fat. It's genetic."

"It's still gross," she retorted, "but I'm glad it's not my fault."

"It certainly isn't."

"Will my lymph system be affected by liposuction?"

"No. Liposuction is superficial. It's done between the fascia of the muscle and the skin. You do get some swelling of the tissue, of course, but your actual lymph system, which is basically the body's drainage system, is affected only to a very small degree. The horror stories you hear are always related to massive liposuction, improperly performed. For someone like you, who's in such good shape, liposuction is a terrific procedure."

"I'm very relieved," Kate said. "I thought I was doing something wrong."

After her liposuction, she was even more relieved to have trim thighs for the first time in her life.

Melinda, age forty-seven, came to see me about having liposuction on her hips. "But everyone says don't do it, because I'm going to die, because it's so risky," she said.

"For you, liposuction wouldn't be risky," I explained. "Your weight is normal, you work out several times a week, and you're fit and healthy. Your legs and belly are both in good shape. To get the shape you desire, you just need a bit of fat taken from your backside.

"You're actually a great liposuction candidate," I went on, "provided that it's done in the right setting, and not too much is taken out. I'd do it here, in my office operating room, with sterile instruments and the greatest care. I can never, as a surgeon, say that nothing can go wrong," I added. "You can die from an allergic reaction to novocaine in the dentist's office. But we do your blood work, we check your EKG, we do everything that is reasonable, because we don't want to miss anything. I will have a board-certified anesthesiologist taking care of you. I think we cover all the bases. The likelihood of your having a serious problem is never zero, but it is close to zero."

"My sister is a nurse, and she said people die from liposuction. She told me to go to Jenny Craig or Weight Watchers instead."

"I agree that people who need to lose weight should diet, not have surgery. An ethical surgeon won't perform elective surgery on anyone who's seriously overweight to begin with. But liposuction is perfect for someone like you, who exercises yet still can't get rid of certain pockets of fat."

Melinda heaved a sigh of relief. "I'm ready to go," she said. "And I won't tell my sister about it until I have nice thin thighs."

If someone who isn't right for liposuction wants the procedure, he or she is rejected. One case was so extreme it was almost funny. George had a huge belly and skinny legs. He looked like he drank three six-packs a day. When he came into my office to discuss liposuction, I told him I'd be glad to do it, but he would have to lose a great deal of weight first, as his body could not handle the anesthesia. I'd be happy to talk with him again when his weight was normal and he was in general good health. I hope he didn't go someplace else, to some doctor who was short on business that week, because he was a disaster waiting to happen.

Certain areas of the body pose more of a challenge than others. Carina, age thirty-six, a patient who'd previously had some liposuction done on her belly, came back because she was unhappy with some of the fat around her waist and back. I told her that those were tough areas because of the nature of the fat.

"I think this can be done, but I do want to be absolutely straightforward that it's more difficult because the fat is more fibrous in this part of the body," I told her. "In your case, I'd probably take out about four to five pounds."

Carina said she thought that having a bit of fat taken off would help her commit even more seriously to exercising and dieting. I often hear that.

"I do watch what I eat and I do exercise," she said. "But I have a new boyfriend, and I have gained a little weight. It's depressing always to watch what you eat, and it's hard to turn those ten pounds back. This will be a renewed incentive to get back to it all."

When I saw her a few months later, she was admiring her new figure. "You took out five, and I lost ten more pounds," she said, beaming. "It was the perfect incentive for me to lose weight."

"That happens to a lot of my patients," I replied. "What I do is good for the economy."

"You go down a dress size and have to buy a whole new wardrobe."

Some women come in wanting a little bit of liposuction in several places. Marsha, who was thirty-six, admitted that she'd gained some weight since her wedding—not an uncommon occurrence—and that she needed help. The weight was evenly distributed, and she was still fit and trim. I told her that liposuction could correct some of her contour problems, but that I couldn't remove all ten pounds she wanted to lose.

"The success of liposuction depends on the elasticity of your skin," I told her. "The better it is, the better your results. Which is why surgeons often joke that an ideal liposuction patient is a nineteen-year-old model! Patients also assume that cellulite can be removed with liposuction. Nothing could be farther from the truth. It's just the opposite—liposuction can make it much worse. But I do have certain techniques to minimize the likelihood of adding to the indentation."

"What do you mean?" she asked.

"I keep the cannula closer to the muscle, rather than closer to the skin, and although that might make you less comfortable for a day or two, it's a good way to minimize any indentation problems."

"I see." She opened her gown and I examined her thighs. "I was thinking about the outer thighs."

"Yes, I could do that."

"I think the hips too."

"And I would recommend your medial, or inner, thighs, just a little bit here," I told her. "The lateral, or outer, thigh is the most common area I do. Women get fat deposits here. Men get love handles instead." I looked even more closely. "You do have a little irregularity on your thighs. I guess we would refer to it as cellulite."

"I guess we would!" she said with a laugh.

"But on your belly, there is almost no likelihood of producing further cellulite," I said. "The chance of your needing another procedure, which we call a secondary, is relatively high, about twelve percent. That's the national statistic. It's because liposuction is not an exact science.

"I'm just being honest," I went on. "It's better to be conservative, to risk the need for a secondary procedure, than to go too far and be unable to correct a problem. If I have to make a decision whether to take more fat or take less, the answer is obviously take less. I can always go back. The risk of taking too much fat the first time is significant. If the skin becomes unbalanced or lumpy, fat grafts would be necessary. This involves harvesting fat from one part of your body and injecting it into another, and that is complicated, because the fat cells don't always live where they're injected, and you might have to keep up the injections until they take. So, yes, my approach is conservative, but I think it's the right approach." If a secondary procedure were needed, I told her, it could often be done with only a local anesthetic.

"Given all that, will it be worth it when it's done?" She looked dubious.

"I think you would get a great improvement. You have your age going for you."

"What about complications?"

"There's the possibility of infection and of hematoma, a collection of blood under the skin, which is rare in liposuction," I said. "If you did have a hematoma, I might have to aspirate it with a needle. There's also a risk of a seroma, which is a collection of fluid, and if that occurred I would have to aspirate too."

"Are the scars really visible?"

"No. The incisions don't leave any noticeable scars, because I put them in your body's natural creases."

"How badly will it hurt? Be honest with me." She looked anxious.

"It's hard to say. Some patients are just, boom, up and around like nothing happened. Others feel like it's the end of the world. Whichever patient you turn out to be," I said, "my staff and I will guide you through the process and give you whatever help you need.

"The two guarantees I give are, one, that I will do the best I can, and two, if there is a problem, I will take care of the problem. I don't operate and run away and have one of my associates take care of you. If I'm out of town, another plastic surgeon covers for me. But don't worry—I don't do surgery and then run to the airport."

"Can you do it here?" she asked, looking a little less skeptical.

"I think it's more comfortable. There is nothing wrong with the hospital, but I think we can take care of you better than anybody. We have six people here. I don't think you'll find a ratio of six caretakers for one patient at any hospital in the world. Nothing beats personalized care. And even if I'm doing some paperwork in my office, I'm only forty feet away from you."

Marsha brightened even more and went to see Lorraine to talk about prices and schedules.

For the right candidate, liposuction can be done with other procedures, as part of a general body sculpting. One of my patients felt that
her body was far too masculine—she wanted more of an hourglass figure. I did liposuction on her waistline and then performed a face-lift and
a tummy tuck, and she was thrilled with the results.

Liposuction is a far less invasive procedure than a tummy tuck, but in
some cases, only a tummy tuck is the right approach. Sara, for instance,
came to me after giving birth to four children. At forty-three, she
weighed only 110 pounds, had no medical problems, and didn't smoke
cigarettes.

When I saw her in her gown, it was hard to believe she needed any
work done. But when she opened it and relaxed her belly, it jutted out
surprisingly far for such a thin woman. It had been stretched so much by
childbirth that no amount of exercising would ever be able to change it.

"You need a tummy tuck, to get rid of the redundant skin and a little
bit of fat," I said. "I'll make the incision where your cesarean incision
was, and I'll do a vertical belly button, rather than a transverse. You'll
bring in a bathing suit, so I can keep the incision marks inside your
bikini line. That way, none of the scar will show, even when you're at the
beach."

"That sounds great," Sara said.

"I'll also do a little bit of liposuction to improve the contour, and
tighten your muscles, because it's not only the skin that's been stretched
out but the fascia as well. I use absorbable sutures, so nothing has to be
removed when the scar is healed. I think that gives a better scar in that
area."

"Do I have to go to the hospital?"

"Yes, you do. Although many surgeries are now done in my office, this
one isn't. I routinely do tummy tucks in the hospital under general anesthesia, but it can be done on an ambulatory basis, and you should be
able to leave the same day.

"It *is* major surgery, in the sense that I undermine, or loosen, a great
deal of skin," I added. "I need to lift your skin away from the muscle all
the way up to your rib cage."

Her husband, who'd accompanied her to the consultation, said he thought that she would probably have to spend the night in the hospital. "Sara and anesthesia don't mix," he explained. "It makes her hyper."

Sara nodded. "For some reason I can't sit still. That's a very annoying feeling. I keep drinking water to get it out of my system."

Patients have very different reactions to anesthesia, and their reactions are very hard to predict. "We'll see how you do and hope you don't have any adverse reactions," I said. "Recovery after a tummy tuck should be easier than recovery after a C-section, because I don't actually cut muscle. But bear in mind that it's a big operation, yet a positive operation. You'll need antibiotics to prevent infection. And I'd be lying if I said there'd be no postoperative pain. I'll prescribe adequate pain medication, and don't hesitate to use it if you need it. I don't want you to suffer."

After the surgery, someone would have to pick her up, because she couldn't drive by herself. She'd come to see me the morning after surgery. Three or four days later, she'd come back and I'd take out the drains.

"I know the drains aren't pleasant, but they are important," I said. "If fluid collects under the skin I have to aspirate it, and I prefer not to do that. No showers are permissible while drains are in. Only a sponge bath."

Her husband, without saying it directly, asked how long she would be unable to care for the house and their children.

"You should get someone for a week," I told him. "Especially because you have toddlers." I turned to Sara. "It's extremely important that you not pick up your little ones. Absolutely no lifting of anything heavy, not even a grocery bag. It'll be about four weeks before you'll be back to your regular routine."

Bonnie was another tummy tuck candidate. At fifty-four, she'd finally lost 150 pounds after sticking to a low-carb diet for nearly two years. She was ecstatic with her discipline and weight loss, but not with her huge folds of excess skin. No matter how elastic the skin is, after a large weight loss it cannot contract to be completely smooth. Bonnie needed a tummy tuck, and she also wanted a face-lift, her breasts lifted, and her arms and thighs made more shapely.

Bonnie now weighed only 130 pounds, and it was hard to imagine her as obese. In her street clothes, she was attractive and vivacious. When she changed into a gown and revealed her thighs, stomach, her breasts, she looked decades older. Her skin was covered in stretch marks and hung in folds like a shar-pei's face. Her breasts sagged so badly that her nipples nearly reached down to her waist. Bonnie was so mortified by her droopiness that she rarely exposed anything other than her face, calves, and hands. Not only that, she was frustrated by the inability to show off and enjoy her newly thin body.

She needed two operations, six months apart. The first would tackle her tummy, breasts, and face, and the second her arms and thighs. Each would take up to six hours. I warned her that she would have long white scars from the arm and thigh reduction that some women would consider unacceptable. Her tummy tuck scars would be hidden in her bikini line.

When she heard that, Bonnie's husband, who was sitting close, holding her hand, paled a little. She merely shrugged. She was determined. It meant the world to her to be able to wear a sleeveless shirt and shorts, and the thought of scars didn't faze her in the least.

"I'll do everything in the hospital," I told her. "And you should stay overnight. It's a fair amount of surgery, done under general anesthesia. I don't like to push the envelope when it comes to my patients. I'm too old for that. I want to go home and sleep like a baby, knowing that everyone is okay."

One day would be plenty in the hospital, and it would make sense to leave as quickly as possible. Being stuck in a hospital bed can actually work against a positive recovery, because one of the most important things to do is to get up and walk.

"If you're not moving your legs, you can get clotting in your calves, which can go to your lungs and result in a pulmonary embolism," I explained. "To protect against that, you'll be wearing special compression garments on your legs during surgery that will prevent formation of clots. But it's also important to become mobilized as soon after the surgery as possible."

Bonnie was anticipating no problems. She even had airline tickets for a long-planned trip with her son a week after surgery, and she hoped it wasn't a problem.

"Everybody's different and I can never give an exact answer, but routinely at that point you should be fine to travel," I said. "You can pretty much do everything except heavy lifting after one week. The real limitations come from the tummy tuck. After surgery, you'll have drains taking any excess fluid out of your abdomen and breasts. They'll come out a few days later. You've already had two cesarean sections and an appendectomy, so you know the drill."

"Can you do anything about my belly button? It's way too low now," she said.

"I'm going to give you a new one," I said.

"And my doctor keeps insisting that I have a hernia."

"No problem. If you do, I'll fix it when I'm in there."

I gave her final instructions. "Don't take any aspirin or aspirin-containing compounds for two weeks before the surgery and two weeks after, as they can thin the blood and compromise healing. Also stop taking herbal supplements. The night before surgery, don't eat or drink after midnight, but it's fine to have a cocktail earlier in the evening. My staff will give you a prescription for antibiotics and pain medicine that should be filled now, to be used after surgery. On the way to the hospital, take one tablet of the Zofran. It reduces the nausea that often affects patients after general anesthesia."

Bonnie nodded. "I can't wait. My friends have been asking me the most insanely idiotic questions. They're all so curious. All the women are more interested in this than anything else. Even when they pretend they're not."

"Any other questions?" I said.

"Do you know how lucky you are to be working on such a beautiful woman?" Bonnie's husband asked.

"You're so right. She's already perfect," I said.

Fourteen

MEN REALLY ARE DIFFERENT

MEN BLEED MORE. THEIR SKIN IS TOUGHER THAN WOMEN'S SKIN, WHICH makes it harder to work with. Worse, they're not as likely to follow instructions for taking care of themselves either before or after their surgery. Combine this with a threshold for pain far inferior to that of women, and you have an instant recipe for endless complaining.

Their wives and girlfriends call them big babies. I, of course, have to be diplomatic, even when my male patients are being amazingly big babies. It comes with the territory.

Most plastic surgeons prefer not to operate on men. They can't take the whining.

That said, male patients—and I've had plenty—come in for everything from liposuction to face-lifts to facial reconstruction after skin cancer surgery. Some of them have even become my friends. Arthur Brandt, who came to my office when I was just starting out after he'd cut his face on a glass door, has been one of my closest friends ever since. A former doctor who now invests in real estate and collects art, he is a big part of my life, in no small part because of the conversations we have about aesthetics and art.

Many of my male patients love to talk about anything having to do with wheels. I don't mind, as I love driving, and it helps relax them during what can be an awkward or difficult consultation. One of my car-loving, speed-loving patients, Carl, was typical of male plastic surgery patients. In his early fifties, active and fit, he came in for a face-lift and a brow-lift. Like a lot of men, he didn't want to look his age.

Like a lot more men, he didn't want the process to inconvenience him in any way whatsoever.

Everything was fine immediately after the surgery, but about a week later he came in with a problem: his forehead was swollen and red. He looked awful.

"What happened?" I asked as I examined him carefully.

"I can't figure it out myself," he said. "The day before yesterday someone said to me, 'Your forehead's a mess. It's getting red.' Now it's on fire."

"You have an infection there."

He nodded. "I figured that's what it was. It just sort of happened quickly. There was some swelling, but it wasn't sore. I thought that was just normal stuff."

"It's probably a suture abscess," I said. "I'll open it up and clean it out. You didn't hit your head or anything, did you?"

"I could have," he admitted.

Typical male answer.

I knew I wasn't going to find out what really had happened. I was sure he'd been doing something he wasn't supposed to.

Fortunately, the infection wasn't bad. I didn't find any pus, only some fluid.

"Things look good," I told him. "It's nothing serious. Please keep taking your antibiotics. You need to apply Bacitracin there too. Use warm compresses three or four times a day."

"What are you, nuts?" he said. "In my spare time?"

I laughed. I knew even as I was saying it that, unlike most women, there was absolutely no chance that Carl was going to follow my directions and actually use the compresses.

Still, it turned out okay, and when I saw him a few months later, he'd healed without a hitch.

Luckily.

Men are less likely to follow instructions before surgery too. During our consultations—and there are always at least two before surgery—I tell all my patients exactly what they should do both before and after the procedure. In addition, Lorraine gives all patients written preoperative instructions. There is really no excuse to forget or become confused. And we always encourage patients to call at any time if they have questions. Because many of them do, I know that we're not an intimidating office and that they really do feel free and comfortable to call me.

The directions patients receive are fairly standard, although there are specifics that vary from patient to patient. As I've said already (and can never say enough!), two weeks prior to surgery, smokers should stop smoking. Everyone should stop taking aspirin, vitamin E, and all herbal supplements one week before and one week after the surgery, due to the possibility that any of them will enhance bleeding. All patients are instructed to have a preoperative screening and medical clearance including a chest X-ray and a complete blood workup. I don't want any surprises in the operating room.

But I was in for a big surprise the day I worked on Jim, who was fifty-three. His surgery would take several hours, as he was having a brow-lift, a face-lift, and some liposuction on his chest. The minute I opened up his face, I knew that I was going to have a problem. He started bleeding and never stopped. I was constantly stanching the flow, but I didn't catch all of it. He bled all over the table, the nurse, the anesthesiologist, my scrubs, my white clogs. He was never in any danger, or I would have stopped the surgery. Yes, men bleed more, but Jim's bleeding was excessive.

During one of our follow-up consultations, I pressed him—nicely, of course—for an explanation. He finally confessed that he'd been taking testosterone pills.

"But they're not herbs, and they're not aspirin," he protested. "So I thought it would be okay."

Never mind that I'd asked him several times if he was taking *any* medications.

Men also find it hard, if not impossible, to slow down after surgery so they can recuperate and heal properly. Many of my female patients work at demanding, high-powered jobs, but they're willing to rest after surgery. Men can be a real pain about it.

Take Greg. He was the senior executive in a very large company. I did a face-lift on him in my office operating suite in the morning, and he came to about an hour later. I went back to check on him as soon as he was stirring.

Greg had just had serious surgery. So what was he doing? Sitting there on the phone, barking instructions to his assistant. His wife was just about tearing her hair out.

This was not the time to be diplomatic. "I'm going to rip that phone right out of your hands if you don't hang up right this instant," I said.

He shrugged but hung up the phone.

I told him that he had to obey my instructions and give up control of his empire for at least two days.

Greg grumbled, but I finally got through to him. His wife later sent me a thank-you note.

He wasn't the only one. After I did a face-lift on Sean, a Wall Street lawyer—a naturally hyperactive master of the universe sort—I gave him the big lecture about how he had to take it easy. He told me he understood.

A day after the surgery, I called him to see how he was doing. He wasn't home. I called his office, trying to keep my temper in check, and his assistant told me he'd been running all over the place. When I finally reached him on his cell phone, he was out voting.

"But it's Election Day!" he said.

"If you don't stop doing what you're doing right this minute, you're going to have a huge problem," I said in my you're-in-trouble voice used for small children and noncompliant male patients. He apologized. He said I was right and he'd go right home.

I called him at home the next day. Thankfully, he answered. He even sounded sheepish. So I knew he really was listening to me.

For about five minutes.

Of course, I understand this Superman ethos. I have a hernia that needs attending to, but I've been putting it off and putting it off. Who has time to have surgery? Not me.

On the other extreme is the guy who wishes he still had Mom around to take care of him. Having a nose job seems to be especially hard for the male of the species. When a man comes in for a rhinoplasty, the first thing my staff asks him is, "How are you when you have a cold?" If he replies that he hates having a cold and it makes him act like a monster, then we know what to expect. Because after you have a rhinoplasty, you feel as if you have a terrible cold. You feel as if you can't breathe, and your nose is extremely swollen. Anyone who has trouble with head-cold symptoms is going to have trouble after the surgery.

I tell this to all my patients, especially the male ones. Do they listen? Are you kidding?

I'll never forget Walter. He was forty-two, a tall, good-looking man, who had a really big nose. I explained the procedure and how he would feel afterward, and he said, as most men do, "Don't worry, I'll be a good patient."

His definition of being a "good patient" was to call the office every day for ten days after his surgery. He usually was satisfied talking to the nurse but once or twice I had to get on the phone. He whined and complained that he felt so congested, he just couldn't breathe. We kept telling him to take Sudafed for the congestion and to drink apple juice to relieve the dryness of the mouth. We kept telling him to put Bacitracin ointment inside the nose and to use a saline spray whenever he felt the need for irrigation.

We told him this over and over. But still he called. And called and called.

One of my most impressive patients was Patrick, a young man who'd lost more than 150 pounds. Even after that achievement, he was still slightly overweight. He had surprisingly good skin quality, though, so I was able to do some liposuction on the parts that he couldn't seem to improve through diet and exercise. I also did a tummy tuck, or abdominoplasty, because the skin hanging down on his belly couldn't possibly be improved through exercise.

Unlike many of my male patients, Patrick was dedicated to looking better, and he always followed instructions. He came to see me three months after the initial procedures to talk about having more.

"I just started going to the gym three weeks ago," he said. "That's when you said I could. But lifting more than light weights hurts like hell."

I told him that wasn't surprising and he shouldn't worry about it. During the abdominoplasty, I tighten the fascia, the covering of the muscle. That can be felt during any straining.

"Oh, that's a relief," he said. "I thought I was doing something wrong. If I don't work out, I'm terrified I'm going to get fat again."

I examined his scars and told him they were coming along well. He should keep applying Spectragel, the ointment I recommend to diminish scars, on them.

"I don't use it much," he said. Of course not. He might be more compliant than most, but he's still a man. "And it's starting to itch here."

"Use the gel regularly. It can really help."

"What about my back? Can I have more liposuction there?"

I'd originally told him that if he felt that he needed more done, he could have additional procedures six months after the initial ones, when he was totally healed.

I examined him carefully. "Looking at you now, I think that does make sense, but keep on exercising as much as you can tolerate. The lower your weight, the better the results."

"I'm doing as much as I can," he said.

"That's great. I wish more of my male patients were like you." He positively glowed. "If you keep on working out and don't firm up, we'll do liposuction."

"My arms still suck too," he admitted. "Can you fix them?"

"I think you have to do the best you can with weights for now. The problem with arm surgery is the scars are pretty alarming. It's not what I'd recommend for you right now. We can talk about it in the future."

Being overweight at a young age can haunt people for a long time, because even after a large weight loss, the body finds it difficult if not impossible to return to a totally normal shape. Stan came to see me about a brow-lift when he was fifty, but he made it clear that he'd been wanting to do something about his breasts for years. Although he was no longer overweight, his breasts were much bigger than he liked.

"This is something that's always bugged me," he said as I took a look at his chest. "As a little kid I was chubby, and even when I was down to my lowest weight, they never went away."

"You're not alone, if that makes you feel any better. Fourteen percent of men have this, so it's not uncommon. Talking about it can be excruciating, I know," I told him. "It's called gynecomastia, and it's a combination of both fat and breast tissue. In the old days we used to put an incision around the areola and do a direct excision with scissors, but for the last twenty years, liposuction is really the only way to go. I make a small incision, just half an inch, on each side of the nipple, in the inframammary fold, and then I infiltrate the area with lidocaine and epinephrine, to stop the bleeding and prevent pain. I have to use a very aggressive form of liposuction because you have both breast tissue and fat. You have no indentations or irregularities, and your skin has pretty good elasticity. You should do very well."

I always ask my patients about the general state of their health, and his recitation was typical.

"I'm fifty," he said. "My cholesterol is a little high, so I take Lipitor. My heart is in good shape. I don't smoke. I'm allergic to penicillin. Sometimes I get stressed. I take an antidepressant, and sometimes I take Ambien when I can't fall asleep."

And because he wasn't at his lightest weight, he wondered whether it would be beneficial to lose a few pounds before the procedure.

"It seems to me that patients who need to lose more than twenty percent of their body weight should do that before surgery, because that's a major loss," I replied. "But in my experience, losing five or ten pounds doesn't make much difference one way or another."

"I don't need to lose twenty. Only about five or ten," he replied.

I nodded. "I know how hard it is to lose weight."

"Is the breast tissue ever going to come back?"

"No. This form of liposuction removes fat cells and glandular tissue permanently. It can't come back. If you were to gain thirty pounds, how-ever, each remaining fat cell would expand—and the idea that you wouldn't gain weight in the part of the body that had liposuction is just a myth. Not every single fat cell is removed, and thus there is still, sadly, room to grow back fat."

After the procedure, he would wear a compression garment around his chest for two weeks to keep down the swelling. I'd prescribe Vicodin for the pain.

"Okay," he said. "Let's talk about my eyes."

Frankly, if Stan hadn't had a problem with his eyelids, I suspect he never would have come to see me in the first place. Gynecomastia is too embarrassing for most men to deal with. But Stan's eyes were a different matter. Dealing with them seemed medically necessary. His lids were extremely hooded and droopy, and he felt they got in the way of his work.

"You have a lot of excess skin on your upper eyelids, although your lower lids are fine," I said after studying his eyes. "If you completely relax your eyelids, the skin comes down and is almost resting on your lashes. At the same time your brow is a little bit down. You're constantly lifting your eyebrows because you want to open up your field of vision. It's also causing wrinkles, because when you activate your frontalis muscle it causes the transverse lines to form on your forehead."

"I know. It gets tiring."

I studied him even more intently. Over the course of a consultation, the problems become more obvious.

So do the solutions.

"I need to do two things. First, I need to trim the excess skin on your upper eyelids, and then, at the same time, elevate the brow about three millimeters. Some patients have hooding only in the eyelids; for others, it's only the brow. In patients such as yourself, where it's a combination of the two factors, you have to address them both."

"If I go ahead with all the surgery, how long will I be out of work? I'm a dentist, and I'm concerned about getting infections during the course of my work if my open skin is exposed to someone with an illness."

"The skin is closed within forty-eight hours. On day four, I pull the stitches out of the upper eyelids. Within a week the wound is healed," I said. "The staples from the brow-lift are taken out on day seven. Basically, you can go back to work that day. There is no bruising of the forehead. Occasionally you get bruising by the upper eyelids. The liposuction around the nipples requires very little recovery. If it were the only procedure you were having, you could go back to the office after a couple of days." I then explained how the endoscopic brow-lift worked, and Stan thanked me and went to talk to Lorraine.

I was actually glad he'd needed the work done on his eyes and brows—otherwise he could have suffered in silence about his breasts. For years, if not forever.

Men can be especially hard to deal with when it comes to following instructions after reconstructive work, particularly the Mohs procedure done for facial skin cancers. Most are grateful for anything that can be done to keep their faces from being disfigured. But some can't be bothered.

Patients come to me directly after the cancer is excised, so that I can work on their faces before the skin starts to heal. Since the defects are often on the nose or cheek, it takes quite a while for the scars to go away. Swelling often remains even at three months, and complete recovery can take a year.

After surgery on the face, it's essential for patients to keep massaging the affected area with a moisturizer, especially where scars are hard. Hard scars need to be worked and scar tissue broken up physically. I usually tell my patients to use Aquaphor ointment. It's unscented, it doesn't aggravate the skin, and it's inexpensive and available in any drugstore. Patients must also use sunscreen religiously.

Do men listen to this? Do pigs fly?

And of course I always tell my male patients that they must follow up on a regular basis with their dermatologists. I used to do post-Mohs surgery reconstruction without ever showing it to my patients. But now I insist that they look at photographs of similar faces after the cancers have been excised, before I get to work. It may be frightening, but I want them to know what a horrible hole they're going to have in the middle of their face. Scaring them is the only way to make them both appreciate how reconstructive surgery can help them as well as understand why it takes so long to get back to normal, and how crucial it is to listen to what I'm telling them. Healing can be a very long, slow process.

One of my Mohs patients was Ricky, a very successful businessman with an easygoing manner. His cancer had been on his nose. As I cleaned off his incision and put steri strips on after the surgical bandages had come off, I told him about the night that Lorraine and I were going to the opera and dinner, and the car that I'd ordered had been driven by someone who nodded off at the wheel.

"I started screaming at him," I told Ricky. "Actually, I had to hit him in the head, once he started scraping along the parked cars. I don't want to die because he had a rough night."

"If you're going to die, you want to die at your own hands," Ricky said with a wink.

"Or with a good-looking girl," I replied, putting on the last of the steri strips. "You don't need a Band-Aid. Apply Bacitracin ointment twice a day for about two weeks."

"When can I start shaving?"

"In three days, but you can use only an electric razor for about two weeks, on a low setting. The sensation is probably a little bit altered, so be careful. You don't want to hurt yourself."

"Okay. And I have to tell you something," he said. "I got a bill from your office for the surgery. You only charged me forty-five bucks."

Obviously, some digits had been left out by mistake.

"I told everyone that you have the most competitively priced medical practice in the city. It's cheaper than Medicare."

I like a patient with a sense of humor. At least I thought it was a joke.

"Now you're hurting me," I said.

Fifteen

UNHAPPY CAMPERS

THERE ARE TWO KINDS OF UNHAPPY CAMPERS.

Those who are unhappy because they're liars.

And those who are unhappy because they have unreasonable expectations. Often, these unreasonable-expectation unhappy campers don't need a plastic surgeon. They need a good therapist.

Both kinds of unhappy campers can make a plastic surgeon's life hell. Still, liars are easier to deal with. That's because I expect patients to lie. They do it all the time. Sometimes their lies are trivial and don't matter in the grand scheme of things. But sometimes their lying can put them in terrible jeopardy.

As you know, I always tell patients to stop taking any drugs that can thin their blood, such as aspirin, and to stop taking all herbal supplements, because we don't always know the effect they may have, one week prior to surgery. If they take any prescription drugs known to pose risks in surgery, I ask them to stop them, too, as long as it's safe. If they smoke, I strongly encourage them to stop two weeks before and after surgery. Smoking definitely interferes with healing, and scars are worse in people who smoke.

Even though I tell this to patients—and emphasize it and repeat it and remind them again and again—patients still manage on a surprising number of occasions to "forget" to stop taking supplements and drugs.

Drug complications are a real issue. Patients who take diuretics, for instance, may have low potassium levels, and that can be a hazard during surgery. Antidepressants can also have a huge effect. One patient's surgery had to be halted halfway through because she hadn't told me that she was taking Elavil, an antidepressant. She was in her early sixties and overall in good health. I had numbed up her face and chin for a face-lift, a blepheroplasty on her eyelids, and a chin implant. As soon as I gave her an injection of epinephrine, her blood pressure soared to 172/95. The anesthesiologist treated her to stabilize the pressure, but it kept veering out of control. I managed to do her upper eyelids and put in the chin implant, but I wasn't about to do her face-lift. I didn't want to make large incisions with her blood pressure so high, because it would mean more bleeding—and potentially a dangerous amount.

I sometimes wonder whether patients think I warn them about surgical risks just to be autocratic, as if it doesn't matter to their health. One of my other warnings about surgery is to not eat or drink after midnight. Once, for a gynecomastia on a twenty-two-year-old man, we started at seven-thirty in the morning, as usual. As he was just starting to be put to sleep, he started vomiting massive amounts of ground beef. I asked him when the last time was that he ate. He said that at ten minutes before midnight he had eaten Cheerios and milk and hamburgers and french fries. We couldn't continue with the surgery, because he couldn't be put under—when patients are vomiting, they can inhale food into their lungs.

And die.

From that charming pile of digested hamburger, I learned that I have to be even more specific with patients. I can't take anything for granted. Now I say: Don't have a big meal at midnight. If there's food in your system, you can throw it up during surgery.

And die.

Herbal medicines are an increasing problem for surgeons. Patients self-medicate, not thinking that herbs are *drugs*. Saint-John's-wort, for example, commonly taken for mild forms of depression, can alter the blood pressure under anesthesia, and people have died as a result. Other herbal treatments can affect clotting, as can vitamin E.

A more difficult problem stems from herbs and supplements containing mystery ingredients. Half the time you don't know what's really in those pills, as the herbal supplement industry isn't regulated by the FDA. My patients are remarkably cavalier about taking these pills. They often don't take them on the advice of an expert, but because their friends are taking them, or a clerk in the health food store recommended them. Nor do they ask my advice about it.

If they trust me to cut their faces open, you'd think they'd want to know my opinion about their self-medicating.

But they don't.

I did a face-lift once on a Russian physician. She ordered an herbal syrup from Russia that was supposed to help the scars. Instead she got a huge allergic reaction that nearly left her with permanently disfiguring scars. Another patient started taking steroids after a face-lift because her girlfriend told her to. That only succeeded in slowing down the healing.

Patients don't lie only to me. I had one not long ago who lied to her husband about how much work she was having done—she told him only her upper lids. When he came to take her home, he was stunned because she looked like she'd been in a boxing match. That's what most patients look like after a full face-lift, brow-lift, and blepharoplasty. He realized that he couldn't take care of her, so she had to wait in my office recovery room for a few hours until we could line up a private duty nurse at the last minute. All because she couldn't tell her husband the truth.

Many patients lie about their age. They leave the birth dates off of their records. This is incredibly stupid, because there's a medical purpose to that question. Anyone over sixty is required to have a thorough evaluation by an internist, as well as a stress test. That's critical to their well-being.

I guess they'd rather lie about their age and die during surgery than have me know they're over sixty-five. As if it matters to me!

Smokers tend to be chronic liars. They want to stop smoking, but they can't. So they lie. But lying about smoking only hurts them, not me. It seriously impedes healing, and the scars never look as good even when they are healed as they look on nonsmokers.

One patient, Fran, was a heavy smoker. Instead of coming in to have her sutures taken out, she went out on the town smoking and drinking and partying. Naturally, her wound didn't heal correctly. She had to have a scar revision, which means that the scar is cut out, the skin is undermined a bit so that it needn't be stretched in order to close, and then it is sewn. Sewing without tension is the key to getting a good scar.

Did she stop smoking after that? Of course not.

Beth was another patient who wouldn't follow directions. She came for a tummy tuck, and as usual I told her to stop smoking, as I tell everyone to stop smoking. She said she did, but she was lying. As a result, she lost a bit of skin at the very end of the scar, near her hipbone. It just wouldn't heal. We had to arrange for visiting nurses because Beth wouldn't change the dressing. She was completely noncompliant. She even stopped keeping her appointments. Our receptionist would call her and say, "You can't do this to yourself. You're hurting yourself. You're going to get infected." She still didn't come back, so I sent her a certified letter saying that if she didn't come to see me she would be compromising her care. I always get suspicious when a patient chronically cancels follow-up appointments or doesn't come back, and I have to do that to protect myself. Sure enough, I got served with legal papers filed by Beth's lawyer. But nothing came of it. She disappeared for good.

I hope that her scar healed properly. But I doubt it.

My mother-in-law had a similar problem with her smoking. I did her eyes, and then her face and brow. I told her she absolutely had to stop smoking two weeks before surgery. The day after her operation, I went to the hospital to check on her and she wasn't in her bed. The bathroom door opened and a cloud of smoke appeared.

I couldn't believe it.

She had the same problem healing. She had to do wet soaks on her scars for months and months, all because she couldn't stop smoking for a month.

On another patient, I did a nasal reconstruction, and the result was absolutely perfect. When I removed the sutures, I could see that her healing was progressing normally. But then she started smoking, and part of her skin didn't heal—it turned a hideous shade of black. I ended up having to perform painful skin grafts on her.

Aside from smoking, one of the stupidest things a patient can do is to fail to keep the follow-up appointments. You can change the course of a scar by keeping an eye on it and jumping right in with appropriate treatment if it's not healing well. There are options like Kenalog, a substance that helps soften certain types of scars; or silicone gel, which prevents scar formation; or lasers, which can be used to flatten raised scars.

But you can't do any of that if the patients disappear.

You wouldn't believe some of the excuses I hear from people who show up weeks or months after they're supposed to. Anything from I was away on business, to I was getting married, to I missed my flight, to the really absurd, I couldn't get a cab.

Okay, enough about liars. Let's move along to the all-too-common unhappy camper with unrealistic expectations.

Patients look at pictures in magazines and see flawless, wrinkle-free skin. They don't understand that even with plastic surgery, no one—not even the most beautiful models or actresses in the world—looks like that in real life, in natural light. Magazine photos are touched up, and then touched up again on a computer that magically erases every conceivable flaw. It's impossible to compete with the flawlessly computerized and retouched images we see every day.

But a lot of my patients don't want to hear that.

Before surgery, I try to show patients, by manipulating their skin and drawing on their photographs, what they will look like afterward. But there's no way they can know exactly what will happen, because there are many things over which I have no control. There are certain limitations: the tissue you are working with, the quality of the skin. With the same procedure on women of identical ages and weight, one will get an excellent result and one will get just a good one. It's impossible to predict every aspect of an outcome, especially with liposuction, which is a less precise form of surgery.

Luckily, the overwhelming majority of my patients are happy.

But there's happy, and *really* happy.

And then there's unhappy, and *really* unhappy.

Sometimes, patients mildly express their disappointment and then get on with their lives. Others get very angry when their postsurgical faces don't match the mental picture they'd envisioned when they first came to see me.

Nina came to me about six months after her face-lift, looking far, far better than she had before surgery. Although she was only in her mid-forties, she'd appeared at least a decade older prior to surgery, because her skin had been ravaged by sunbathing and smoking.

When I walked into the examining room she was friendly and we had our usual banter, but I could feel waves of her frustration and hostility.

"I'm just not happy with it here," she said, holding her palm to her jawline. "It's still slack, and I don't understand why. My girlfriend went to a different surgeon, and she looks great. With me, I don't think there was that much of an improvement."

I let her talk. I knew she wanted to vent. And what could I say? That you came to me with really horrible skin, and that your girlfriend had probably started out in better shape? No. I would never, ever say such a thing to a patient.

Even though it was the truth.

"I see," I said.

"And there's still a scar."

"That will get better."

"Well, I don't like it. I just don't think it looks good here. When I tell people I had a total face-lift, they say, 'Well, what happened here?'" she went on, running her hand under her chin again.

"If this really bothers you, I can open up the incision and tighten it. Or I can do laser all the way around and go even deeper around the creases. Either one will make it better, but neither will make it perfect," I told her, then called Lorraine. Nina needed to see how much better she looked, and that was easy enough to do with her "before" photographs.

"You know, you have to think about whether it will be worth undergoing another procedure. This area will look better, but it's not going to be completely smooth."

"But you admit that it needs a little tweaking."

"I think it's reasonable to do," I said diplomatically. "But it is a procedure."

Lorraine arrived with the photos and showed them to Nina, who frowned and pushed them away. She was clearly so frustrated by her jawline that she chose not to see the extent of her improvement.

"I think it would be reasonable to start initially with only the laser and see if you get enough improvement with it," I suggested.

Her frown deepened. She seemed clearly displeased with the idea. "Laser hurts a lot, right? To be quite honest, that face-lift was a piece of cake. I wasn't even black and blue." Then she asked more questions about the recovery time, and the risk, and where the scar would be.

I explained that surgery is more of a stress on the body, but in some ways the recovery is easier. Laser takes many weeks to heal, although after one week you can put on camouflaging makeup.

"It's easier for you just to have the laser. It's straightforward. Because it's easier for you, my tendency is to go with that first. We always have the more drastic surgical option later. For that, I'd use twilight sleep and do the procedure here in the office. But you'd still need a private duty nurse for the first night."

At that point, her frown disappeared and she seemed happy enough with my suggestions. She air-kissed me good-bye, but I couldn't tell what she would decide to do. Later, Lorraine told me that when informed that there would be a $1,200 operating room fee and a separate fee for the anesthesiologist, Nina got really annoyed.

"Do you think that's fair?" Nina argued. "He should have done it the first time. When I came back after the surgery, the nurse said we missed a little."

"He didn't miss anything," Lorraine said. "The nurse was wrong."

Nina told Lorraine she was happy with her eyes but not with her neck. Lorraine told her that there was only so much I could have done in one procedure without her having serious problems later. That she had to look at her skin texture and existing damage from years of baking in the sun and smoking. Lorraine then added that I wouldn't be charging any fee for my time, but fees had to be paid to the other employees for their time, and that if she did it at the hospital, it would cost far more.

Nina left in a huff, and we never saw her again. She had gotten a good result from her face-lift. She just hadn't wanted to face the truth about the damage she'd done to her own skin. The results of her friend's face-lift were irrelevant to her case.

Plus she wanted more work done for free.

Patients like Nina pinpoint a crucial fact: always err on the side of caution whenever you go in for surgery. While working on a patient, if I can stretch the skin more, or stretch it less, I stretch it less. I do that for a good reason. It's much easier to go back and do a little more than to correct something that turns out to have been a mistake. Many mistakes can never be fixed. Original skin and bone cannot be replaced. Nor can everything always be fixed in one operation. If you pull too tight, with too much tension, the scars are bad. You can pull only so much in one procedure.

Other doctors might have told Nina, "This is your anatomy and this was the state of your skin's elasticity, so these are the results, and I can't do better." But I hate to do that, if there is any possibility of making it better. Doctors in general don't like to do revisions, which we call secondary procedures. But it's an ego thing with me. I want to do the best that can possibly be done. Nina could have gotten a better result with lasers and perhaps a secondary.

But not better enough to make her a happy camper.

Other patients have something go wrong and although they're unhappy, they don't blame anyone. They understand it's just the way it goes. One of my favorite patients, Sylvia, had her breasts augmented three years ago. One day Lorraine got a hysterical call from her. She was in the emergency room of a nearby hospital, where doctors had told her that her implants were infected and they'd have to be removed immediately. I got on the phone and told her to leave the emergency room and come right over.

When she arrived, I took a look at her breasts and knew she had an abscess. Three days earlier, she was treated and given an antibiotic but it wasn't the right one for her problem. I cleaned out the abscess and put her on the right antibiotic, hoping that the infection would resolve and the implants could be saved. But it didn't work. Within forty-eight hours, she was in the hospital on intravenous antibiotics, and I had to remove both implants. She'd gotten the infection from scratching a bug bite, which progressed when it hadn't been treated properly. After the surgery to remove the implants, she healed properly, and six months later, she came back wanting new ones put in. She had so enjoyed having her breasts larger that there was no question in her mind that it was worth trying again, even though, of course, because it was several years after the first surgery, she would have to pay my surgical fee again.

Sometimes results are disappointing to people who didn't need a big change in the first place. Rosalind, an attractive woman of forty-seven, had a laser treatment under her eyes to erase her fine lines, as well as upper and lower blephs to make her eyes less puffy. She came back for her regular follow-up appointment six weeks after the procedure and complained that she wasn't happy with the results. She said she didn't see much difference in how she looked.

Overall, she did look better. But it was admittedly subtle because Rosalind hadn't had a big problem to begin with. It's a tough call. If you do too much to the patient, she looks obviously operated on, and that's not what my patients want. I prefer to be on the conservative side. The downside is too great. If I had damaged Rosalind's skin with laser trying to get a more noticeable result, I could have repaired it only with a complex secondary procedure.

With surgical patients, at least we have the "before" pictures so that people who don't believe they've really changed can look at the proof. The pictures are taken by a professional and show every wrinkle and pore, so there's no need to imagine anything. It's different with injectibles like Botox. It hasn't been worth making people pay for professional photos before injections; the time and the expense would be too daunting. But the increasing use of injectibles has resulted in more unhappy campers complaining. They say the material fell out, or it didn't work. In most cases neither of those things are true. Patients simply can't remember—or don't want to remember—what they used to look like. And of course the changes are much more slight, so there's more likelihood that people will be disappointed. Sometimes they come back asking for another injection, and they don't want to pay for it. They say it's owed to them because the first one failed to deliver.

I don't want to get into fights with patients, but I don't want to be cheated, either. I know that a certain percentage of patients will come in because they want another injection for free. It's not an ideal situation. We try to do the best that we can to have a happy patient.

Sometimes patients are unhappy because they don't realize the importance of follow-up care. They come in frustrated that a scar is not healing as well as they want it to, and then under questioning they admit that they haven't been using the Spectragel I prescribed for softening.

And then there are the *really* unhappy campers.

The kind with a lawyer in tow.

I've rarely been sued, and so far I haven't lost a case. Typically, I was happy with the surgery, and then all of a sudden the papers were served. I knew I hadn't done anything wrong, and I felt completely betrayed. You think it's the end of the world when you get socked with legal papers. The prospect of being sued—and of having to think about the possibility every day—is the only thing I don't like about being a plastic surgeon.

The first lawsuit was filed by a Polish woman, Katya, who came to me after I gave a talk at the Polish consulate. I did her lower eyes and fixed the deviated septum in her nose.

Two years later, I was served with papers. The suit alleged that she couldn't close her eyes, which was irrelevant because I hadn't operated on her upper eyes.

The judge wanted me to settle, because he didn't want to spend four days overseeing the trial. I was outraged and made a speech about how my family escaped from a totalitarian system to have freedom under the law, and I insisted on pursuing my right to trial. Katya's lawyer called "expert" witnesses, who were hardly expert. But there was no problem with her eyes. And even if there had been, they couldn't have been caused by the surgery I did. The jury deliberated for all of seven minutes. I was exonerated.

Another lawsuit was filed by a patient named Vanessa, who'd had dermabrasion. She was a beautiful, elegant woman, one of our first patients. We all used to sit and talk on the sofa in the waiting room. She would tell me about her daughter's upcoming wedding, and we would discuss wedding gowns. After the dermabrasion, she healed very nicely. A few months later, however, she developed fever sores around her mouth. I sent her to a specialist for treatment but heard nothing further from her. My office staff called, but she never returned our calls. A few months after that, I got served with a complaint.

Vanessa was suing me because of her inability to kiss her husband. She was asking to be compensated for the mental anguish.

I was mystified, because the dermabrasion had gone well. I couldn't understand why she had gotten an infection, but sometimes it happens. I told my attorneys that she had been told that infection was a risk of surgery. If the surgery had caused the infection, it was not malpractice, just an unfortunate side effect.

It wasn't until the final deposition, shortly before trial, that her attorneys found out that Vanessa's fever sores and infection were, in fact, due to an entirely unrelated virus she had contracted. The suit was promptly dropped because she didn't want to have to testify in court about her herpes.

Although I was successful in these cases, the economic cost was sky-high. My malpractice carrier had to spend money defending me. Last year, I paid $55,000 in malpractice insurance. I'll be paying even more next year. My carrier has to raise its rates to keep up with the ludicrous number of frivolous lawsuits filed by unscrupulous attorneys. That cost is passed along to you, the patient, in the form of higher fees to cover my overhead.

Worse, these frivolous lawsuits take valuable court time away from the truly heinous malpractice suits that deserve to be filed for patients who've been permanently injured or disfigured or killed.

When I read stories of shoddy work and suffering patients, I get frustrated and furious, because of the harm done to the innocent and because of the way it reflects badly on all the competent surgeons in my field.

I have only once testified as an expert witness in a malpractice case, because it's nearly impossible for me to take the time away from my practice. Occasionally, though, I hear of something a doctor has done that is so egregious that I feel compelled to take action.

In one case, the woman's face was maimed for life. During a face-lift on this woman, her doctor dissected in the wrong plane and killed every single nerve on her face. She will forever have a distorted face. On one side there is simply no expression, so she looks as if she's had a stroke or is partially paralyzed when she smiles. She is no longer able to do anything as simple as squint.

What I found the most infuriating during the trial was that this doctor was not only incredibly annoying and arrogant but also didn't think he'd done anything wrong. A woman can no longer show her true feelings on her face, one of our most important abilities, but it wasn't his fault. Luckily, the jury thought otherwise, and he got the verdict he deserved. In the end, though, the verdict and the money were not enough to compensate this woman for what had been done to her.

That doctor was not well-known or experienced. But the sad thing is that sometimes malpractice is committed by doctors with good credentials, with the right education, with articles to their names, and many other satisfied patients.

All kinds of things can go wrong, as all surgeons know, and in my opinion the fact that doctors now operate in their offices, without hospital staff privileges and outside scrutiny, makes it more difficult to evaluate what actually happened.

For example, a doctor in New York had his license suspended after being accused of botching breast implants and hiding the risks of surgery. The doctor claimed that the other surgeons were just ganging up on him to get rid of a competitor, as he had one of the largest cosmetic surgery practices in his area and advertised widely. One of the many lawsuits against him was filed by a woman who went to him for carpal tunnel surgery but claimed that he pressured her into having a face-lift as well. She finally agreed, but then sued, arguing that he'd made her look deformed. Another patient said he made her breasts way too big, and that liposuction had left her skin lumpy. She described her postsurgical appearance as "like Frankenstein."

Another doctor had a history of drug addiction, and the malpractice suits filed against him claimed that he operated on patients when he was in a stupor. Doctors have easy access to drugs, so addiction is a risk of our job. According to documents in that case, the doctor was injecting himself with propofol, a sedative often used in plastic surgery. And he was doing it while he was seeing patients. Patients suffered infections, scarring, and deformities that sent them to other doctors for corrective surgery.

In another case involving multiple lawsuits, a doctor was charged with malpractice more than a dozen times in a dozen years. The claims ranged from disfiguring a woman with a laser treatment to causing the death of a sixty-six-year-old woman during liposuction. In still another case, a seventy-year-old woman died of respiratory failure after a face-lift; the same doctor treated a forty-nine-year-old woman who died after surgery that included a face-lift, nose job, and eyelid operation. She fell into a coma six hours after the operation and never recovered. The doctor who treated both women alleged that the older woman had been cleared by her internist for surgery, even though she had a blood disorder. The other, he said, happened because a nurse anesthetist gave the patient a narcotic after the surgery to dull the pain without telling him.

Another surgeon lost his license to practice in the United States, so he moved to Mexico and started a practice there—aimed at women from the United States who were looking for less expensive treatments.

Then there was the doctor who settled a lawsuit with a patient after he left a sponge in her buttocks when he put an implant there. The same doctor was investigated in the death of a man during liposuction and a penile implant.

One doctor had his medical license revoked when a liposuction patient bled to death after he took out an unbelievable *nine quarts* of fat during liposuction, and then went on to do a face-lift and a brow-lift. The surgery took more than ten hours, an absurdly long time to work on a patient on the table for elective surgery. The state also took away the anesthesiologist's license.

The moral of the story?

Choose your surgeon wisely. Have realistic expectations. Tell the truth.

Then you won't be an unhappy camper.

Sixteen

THE NEVER LIST: WHAT YOU REALLY NEED TO KNOW AND ASK YOUR PLASTIC SURGEON BECAUSE IF YOU DON'T YOU MIGHT BE SORRY

MORE THAN ANYTHING, I WANT EVERYONE TO UNDERSTAND THAT PLASTIC surgery is serious business. So here's my fifteen plastic surgery commandments, or my never list.

1. NEVER Shop for a Bargain

Sorry, but there is no such thing as a bargain when it comes to plastic surgery. If you go to someone who promises to give you Botox for a third of the price that others are charging, there's a reason.

You'll be getting only a third of the quantity that I'd give you.

Drugs like Botox have a fixed price. Trust me, no one gives anything away.

Same with surgery. If you go to a doctor who charges less, the odds are good that he or she is less qualified or less experienced than someone who charges more.

I'll admit, however, that there are exceptions. You may find a young and extremely talented doctor who's just starting out, and you can benefit by getting a better price from him or her than you would from some-one with more experience. But generally speaking, surgeons with more experience are better because they've seen more and done more. They understand how wounds heal. They know how much skin softens up and goes slack. Plastic surgery is a subtle field whose intricacies can be learned only over the years. It becomes a knack. I'm not trying to be arrogant saying that—I learned it after years of experience. My work now is far superior to the work I did when I first started. Doctors charge for that, simply because they can.

It's your face, your body, and your life. If you can't afford someone good, save your dollars until you can.

Honestly, would you want someone without the deepest possible knowledge and experience slicing off your face or sucking out your fat? I recently saw a woman who'd had a chemical peel at a hair salon in Florida and ended up with a massive, disfiguring scar on her face. No one should get anything but the mildest peel from a salon. I was flabbergasted.

I may not be Einstein, but I would know enough to not go to a hair salon to have chemicals put on my face.

It's up to you to take responsibility for your health and well-being. Plastic surgery is most often elective surgery.

Elect to be smart.

Searching for bargains will most likely cost you triple in the long run. The only one who gets the bargain is the doctor who has to fix the mistakes.

Like me.

It's amazing how irrational some people are in their effort to save a few dollars. A woman came for Botox. She called the next day and wanted information on how and where we ordered it as well as how large a syringe we used. When Lorraine asked her why, she said that her hus-band, who was a podiatrist, was going to inject her with Botox next time. I would have said nothing, because that's my style. But Lorraine doesn't keep her opinions to herself. She told the woman that she was foolish to have a podiatrist—husband or no husband—give her Botox injections.

Her face would end up looking like a foot.

2. NEVER Have Surgery by Anyone Other than a Qualified, Board-Certified, Experienced Plastic Surgeon

Don't pick a surgeon based on an advertisement in a newspaper—much less the subway. Generally, good plastic surgeons don't advertise. Our professional society, the American Society for Aesthetic Plastic Surgery, frowns on this practice.

Ask doctors you trust for recommendations. Choose three surgeons to consult, doctors who you believe are at the top of the field where you live. Then interview them. Write your questions down so you don't forget any. Speak up. You're paying for the doctor's time, and any surgeon worth his or her reputation will be happy to answer anything you ask, no matter how trivial you think it is. Informed, prepared patients make our job much easier.

After the novelist Olivia Goldsmith died during surgery for a chin-lift in January 2004, there was a lot of publicity about her case. The only good thing to come out of it, as far as I'm concerned, was that patients started asking me more questions. One woman in particular asked me a question that I thought was brilliant. I was doing only a minor, laser procedure on her, but she wanted to know whether the kind of doctor who is doing the surgery actually makes a difference. She wasn't asking whether I could do a better face-lift than someone else. She was asking whether the doctor's overall experience would make a difference when it came to saving her life.

Of course, it does. Let's say, hypothetically, that I was doing a breast augmentation, and all of a sudden there was a major catastrophe to this patient in the operating room that necessitated my opening up her chest. Do you want a doctor who has training in that, or do you want a dermatologist who has never seen a chest tube placed in a chest cavity since his or her surgical training rotation in the emergency room twenty-five years before?

God forbid something major happens to you during elective (or any kind of) surgery. But on the minuscule chance that it does, you want the doctor with the deepest surgical experience to be in the room to help you survive.

Sadly, I don't think young surgeons have that kind of training any-more. Now they go directly into training for plastic surgery. They never do trauma cases, or run a service at Bellevue the way I was trained. I'm extremely grateful that I have that knowledge stored away so I can call upon it if I ever need to. I think all surgeons should have it.

Also be sure to ask about the protocol for surgical emergencies.

This protocol extends to the facility where you will be having the sur-gery done. Always make sure that it has the proper licensing and equip-ment. Ask to see the doctor's certificate for the operating room if it is in his or her office. There are reasons for this. In a case not long ago, an eighteen-year-old woman who went to a Philadelphia area doctor for liposuction died not long after the procedure when a clot of fat entered her lungs. There's no way of knowing whether the medical facility lacked something that could have saved her. But during the postmortem inves-tigation, it turned out that the facility wasn't properly licensed.

3. NEVER Have Gore-Tex or Silicone Put in Your Lips

I've taken care of enough problems caused by these materials to know it's not a good idea. Implants made from these permanent substances are too extreme and artificial looking. Worse, removing this material is not easy. It has to be cut out, and that can leave a visible scar and a deformed lip.

4. NEVER Have a Face-Lift Without Asking Where the Incision Will Be

It must be behind the front part of the ear, called a retrotragal. Otherwise the scar will be more obvious. Incision placement is so important you must pay attention to it and ask questions.

5. NEVER Say Yes to a Large Procedure When a Smaller One Can Just as Easily Give You the Result You Want

There are doctors who pull what amounts to an insurance scam by sug-gesting you get a large procedure—perhaps a realignment of the jaw—

rather than a chin implant. They do that because the jaw surgery may be reimbursed by the insurance company as a necessary reconstructive procedure, but the implant won't be. A chin implant isn't anywhere as complicated or painful as a realignment.

6. NEVER Get Breast Implants if Your Mother or Sister Had Breast Cancer

Implants in most cases pose absolutely no problem. But if significant scarring develops, that can interfere with mammography, and cancer might be difficult to detect. There's no way of predicting who will develop scarring, so for people with a high risk of breast cancer, it's not worth the risk.

7. NEVER Get Buttocks Implants

Every single one I've seen, whether presented in real life, photographs, or journals, looks ridiculous. Women appear to have bubbles in their butts.

Besides the fact that they look completely bizarre, there are medical reasons to stay away from this procedure. It's crazy to put a foreign body in a weight- and tension-bearing area. Especially an area like your rear end, which is constantly in motion. The implant will rupture from the pressure, or move, or contract.

But there are always doctors who will do surgeries that really aren't appropriate.

And patients who demand that they're done.

8. NEVER Believe a Doctor Who Says
You Can Have a Face-Lift with Fat Injections

Contrary to many articles written about facial fat injections in women's magazines, I don't believe they really deliver much. And a fat injection can end up giving an awkward look, making you look puffy, distorted, and sometimes, oddly enough, rectangular, especially if it was put into the cheeks and the angle of the jaw. Almost like you're on steroids.

Fat injections are tricky. Sometimes, postsurgery, if you have an indentation, a fat injection can be the best way to fill it. The fat is your own, harvested from your belly or thigh—so there's no worry about being rejected by your body—and then injected where needed. But it's a very imprecise procedure, as many of the fat cells do not reestablish themselves. They simply die.

Which means you have to go through the procedure all over again.

9. NEVER Have a Thigh-Lift Unless Your Inner Thigh Looks Like a Shar-Pei

It leaves a scar that's way too big for most people's taste. Focus instead on the eyes and face, because that's what people see. Having work done there makes the biggest difference in your appearance with the least amount of scarring.

10. NEVER Let a Doctor Talk You into Taking More Than Ten Pounds Off During a Single Liposuction Procedure

It's just too dangerous. It can kill you.

11. NEVER Go Under Without Asking Beforehand What Kind of Anesthesia the Doctor Is Planning to Use

If at all possible, stay away from general anesthesia. It is more traumatic for the body with a longer postoperative recovery. Mistakes can be made. The endotrachial tube can be put in the esophagus rather than the trachea. Patients may also go into laryngospasms where they can't breathe.

I don't think patients realize that I can't harm them in any profound way, but the anesthesiologist can kill them. In all my years of practice, I don't remember a patient ever asking if the anesthesiologists I use are board certified. Nor has anybody ever asked me whether I use an anesthesiologist who has experience with ambulatory surgery, which happens to be critical, because putting somebody to sleep for a gallbladder operation is very different from putting someone to sleep for a face-lift.

You want the very best anesthesiologist working on you, no question about it. If the doctor you're consulting brushes away concerns, give him or her the brush-off and walk out the door.

Also ask whether the surgeon will be administering the anesthesia or whether it will be done by an anesthesiologist or nurse anesthetist. I personally think that the surgeon should do surgery and leave the anesthesia to another doctor who specializes in that field. It can lead to problems if one person does both. Sure, it cuts down on the cost, but is it worth dying for?

12. NEVER Hesitate to Ask What Qualifications the Doctor Has

Find out where he or she trained and with whom. In my opinion, the best places for plastic surgery training are New York University, University of Texas Southwestern Medical Center, and UCLA. Ask whether the doctor ever did a fellowship in aesthetic surgery. The best one is at Manhattan Eye, Ear and Throat Hospital in New York City. There are other good ones, of course, but fellows there receive the greatest exposure to the largest variety of aesthetic surgery cases in America.

In addition, find out whether the doctor is certified by the American Board of Plastic Surgery. Accept no substitutes. Many boards will certify doctors for a small fee, but those certificates don't carry the same weight. There is a facial plastic surgery certification, and a cosmetic dermatology board, but the only meaningful certificate is the one recognized by the American Board of Medical Specialties and the only one relating to plastic surgery with that authority is the American Board of Plastic Surgery.

The other certifications do not represent the same level of training. For example, doctors can attend a weekend course and get a certificate in dermatological surgery. Look carefully at the certificate. In general, the more scummy the organization, the more impressive the certificate.

It's also important to ascertain which procedures the doctor does most often. If a doctor is known for his breast implants, don't go to him or her for a rhinoplasty. You need to get a sense of many specific procedures this doctor has done so you can make an appropriate choice. If a doctor says, "I only do it this way," it tells me he or she doesn't know how to do other techniques and isn't willing to be flexible—and that limits the patient's options.

Also check the hospital privileges. Find out whether the surgeon has privileges at the hospital to do the particular procedure you are going to have done, even if you are having it done in his office. There is peer review in hospitals. There is no peer review in a nonaccredited office surgery facility. I believe that problems are much more likely to develop in nonaccredited surgical facilities.

13. NEVER Just Assume That Your Surgeon Will Actually Be Doing All of the Surgery

Some surgeons do only a portion of the procedure, and it's important to find out beforehand exactly what aspects your doctor will, or will not, be handling. You should also ask whether the doctor will be doing the bulk of the follow-up care. If a patient has a tummy tuck and I examine her the next morning, I can see whether or not there is a hematoma. A resident or a nurse might not recognize it.

You're paying top dollar. The doctor you choose should be the doctor doing all the surgery, and all the follow-up.

14. NEVER Have Surgery Without Seeing the Doctor's Handiwork on Other Patients

If patients ask us for references, we're happy to oblige, and we hook them up with former patients who've had similar surgery. If a doctor claims he or she doesn't have anyone for you to talk to, that's a red flag. Photographs can be altered, retouched, or bought, so it's always best to see the results done on a real, live person.

15. NEVER Ignore Your Gut

If you consult with several doctors who meet all of the important qualifications, who are board certified in plastic surgery, and who have the appropriate training, at the end of the day the choice of which one to hire is completely up to you. There's a certain amount of trust that you have to place in the surgeon. You have to trust your gut that this is the right doctor. As well as the right office. You have to feel comfortable not only with the doctor but also with his or her staff.

Following these steps won't totally protect you from doctors who do an inferior job. There are doctors who are not board certified in plastic surgery—ear, nose, and throat doctors, perhaps, or cosmetic dermatologists—who do good work, and there are board-certified plastic surgeons who do not. Cosmetic dermatologists, for example, often have a remarkably deft hand with injectibles, as they do so many of these procedures. I can only argue for doing as much research as possible.

Do your due diligence and trust your instincts. There are too many people out there who don't look better after plastic surgery. They look *different*, but they don't necessarily look better.

The more research you do, the more you will learn. Aesthetic standards and values vary tremendously. Visual judgment is entirely subjective. There are doctors who proudly show photographs of their handiwork, yet you might look at them and think they're hideous. If the "after" photo doesn't appeal to you for whatever reason, listen to your gut.

And say good-bye.

APPENDIX

There are a number of organizations that can provide information about whether surgeons are board certified in plastic surgery and whether their surgical suites are accredited.

The American Board of Plastic Surgery, Inc. (ABPS), certifies plastic surgeons. To be certified, a doctor must have graduated from an accredited medical school and must have completed at least five years of additional training as a resident surgeon. This includes a minimum three-year residency in an accredited general surgery program and a minimum two-year residency in plastic surgery. To become certified, a doctor then must successfully complete comprehensive written and oral exams. Board certification is a voluntary process. ABPS is one of the twenty-four specialty boards recognized by the American Board of Medical Specialties (ABMS). It is the ony ABMS board that certifies in the full spectrum of plastic surgery. It can be found on the Web at www.abplsurg.org.

The American Board of Medical Specialties (ABMS) can also verify physician certification. Its Web address is www.abms.org.

The American Society of Anesthesiologists (ASA) can offer information about anesthesiologists and can be found on the Web at www.asahq.org.

The American Association for Accreditation of Ambulatory Surgery Facilities (AAAASF) is a voluntary program for inspection and accreditation of medical facilities and is the primary accreditation authority of office-based surgical suites. It is at www.AAAASF.org.

The American College of Surgeons (ACS) is at www.facs.org. The letters F.A.C.S. after a surgeon's name mean that his or her education, training, and competence have passed a rigorous evaluation.

The American Society for Aesthetic Plastic Surgery Inc. (ASAPS), at www.surgery.org, is an association of plastic surgeons who must be board certified in cosmetic plastic surgery by the American Board of Plastic Surgery.

The American Society of Plastic Surgeons (ASPS) provides information on procedures and membership standing of surgeons, who must be board certified to belong. It can be found on the Web at www.plasticsurgery.org.